MUSCULOSKELETAL DISEASES AND *HOMEOPATHY*

LUC DE SCHEPPER, M.D., Ph.D., Lic.Ac., C.Hom., D.I.Hom.

PUBLISHING

FULL OF LIFE PUBL.
PO BOX 31025
SANTA FE, NM 87594

Other books by the same author:

"Acupuncture for the Practitioner," 1985

"Candida, the Causes, the Symptoms, the Cure," 1986

"Peak Immunity," 1989

"Full of Life," 1991

"Human Condition: Critical," 1993

"How to Dine Like the Devil and Feel Like a Saint," 1993

1st printing

Library of Congress Catalog Card Number: 94-071177

ISBN 0-942501-01-2

Printed by Community Press, Provo, Utah

Full of Life Publishing, Santa Fe, NM 87501

Note to Reader and Disclaimer

The information in this book is presented for information purposes only. All therapies, treatments, exercises or energetic interventions of any nature should be undertaken only under the direct guidance and care of a properly and legally, fully trained health care professional specializing in the services rendered. Nothing described in this book should be construed by any reader or other person to be a diagnosis or treatment for any disease or condition. Neither the author nor publisher can accept any responsibility for any ill effects resulting from the use or misuse of the information contained herein. Any uses or misuses of the information presented here for educational purposes are the responsibility of the reader.

Cover and design by Yolanda De Schepper

DEDICATED TO HUMAN SUFFERING

ACKNOWLEDGMENTS

I could not have written this book without the help and understanding from all my patients who have entrusted their care to me. I am greatly indepted to them. I owe a lot to my teacher Robin Murphy, N.D., who has strengthened my love for homeopathy. His generosity in sharing his knowledge is a trademark of only great teachers. And most important, without the support and artistic talents of my beloved wife, Yolanda, this book would not have been possible.

Luc De Schepper, M.D., Ph.D., Lic.Ac., C.Hom., D.I.Hom.

500 N 441

For more info

Visit Web site:

www.drluc.com

"THE REALLY GREAT CREATORS HAVE ALWAYS BEEN MEN OF CHARACTER AND MORAL COURAGE."

TABLE OF CONTENTS

INTRODUCTION

This book is intended for both the beginner and the advanced homeopath. Any physician will benefit from the knowledge contained in this book, since "musculoskeletal diseases and injuries" comprise a large part of patient complaints. This book is especially oriented to the chiropractor, the D.O. and those M.D.s who wish to add valuable knowledge and therapeutic power to their arsenal. This book would be very helpful to acupuncturists, were it not for the fact that most acupuncturists are forbidden to practice homeopathy. I would shortchange the serious-minded layman by not mentioning how useful this book could be for them. After all, some of the greatest homeopaths, Melanie Hahnemann and Von Boeninghausen, were laymen, yet were, according to Hahnemann himself, his best pupils.

I have divided this book into three sections. Section one consists of the Laws and Principles of homeopathy. In it, the practitioner will find all the guidelines he needs to prescribe for and manage the patient. It is of utmost importance and little understood, even by many homeopaths. Although Hahnemann has given us the best book one could ever read, the 6th Edition of the *Organon,* it is my sincere hope that this book will help the physician deal with his patient in an intelligent and efficient way. Following the principles and guidelines expressed in these paragraphs is the ideal.

Section two describes the clinical or musculoskeletal conditions we want to treat. I realize that this is somewhat contradictory to section one, in which I contend that there are no disease names, but only people with diseases. However, I realize too, that it is infinitely easier for the practitioner to begin when he has something familiar to fall back on. What I have done in this book is to make a bridge between Western medicine and homeopathy. Laymen and doctors think in clinical terms and they are apt to select outstanding symptoms and build the remedy around this complaint. Famous homeopaths like Compton Burnett M.D. and George Royal M.D. among others, proceeded in the same fashion. Once the bridge has been crossed, it is my sincere wish that the practitioner, stimulated by his early successes through using this book, would continue to explore the vast world of homeopathy. Only then will he or she comply with Hahnemann's wishes: "*To imitate him, but to imitate him well.*"

Section three is the Materia Medica of the musculoskeletal diseases. Again, I have purposely limited the symptoms and indications to the topic itself. I have added the mental and emotional symptoms of each remedy in light of their importance. And again, the serious student's curiosity should be stimulated by wanting to know the total picture of the remedy. But I believe that putting it in this context is helpful for the busy practitioner. May it inspire many of you to begin to "see the light."

SECTION ONE

GENERAL PHILOSOPHICAL AND THERAPEUTIC HOMEOPATHIC PRINCIPLES

"It is infinitely easier to contradict than to investigate, infinitely easier to sneer at truths and to present them in repulsive light by misrepresentation and falsifications than to devote one's whole life, as Hahnemann did, to the laborious and conscientious search for truth by faithful observation of the nature of things in the most careful trials and applications of their results to the welfare of humanity."

VITAL ENERGY

1. *"In the healthy condition of man, the spiritual force, the dynamism that animates the material body, rules with unbounded sway, and retains all the parts of the organism in admirable, harmonious vital operation, as regards both sensations and functions, so that our indwelling, reason-gifted mind can freely employ this living, healthy instrument for the higher purpose of our existence." "The material organism, without the vital force, is capable of no sensation, no function, no self-preservation; it derives all sensation and performs all the functions of life solely by means of the immaterial being (the vital principle) which animates the material organism in health and in disease."* <u>*Organon*, 6th Edition,</u> 9th and 10th paragraphs, by Dr. Samuel Hahnemann.

   It is amazing that Western medicine had to wait so long to accept the psychosomatic unity. Only since the early '80s, has medicine tried to integrate the mind and emotions into what they called a "new" science, "Psychoneuroimmunology," linking emotional and mental distress to alterations in the strength of the immune system. *"Man is a composite being, a multidimensional entity, a synthetic unity of life, consciousness and intelligence." "Mind is the key to man,"* said Hahnemann 200 years ago, while Dr. James Kent, the famous homeopath from Chicago (†1916) wrote, *"Man consists in what he thinks and what he loves and there is nothing else in man."*

2. A true homeopath, or any practitioner, be it a medical doctor, chiropractor, acupuncturist, hygienist, must realize the concept of *Vital Energy*. Two thousand years ago, the Chinese called it "Chi," the basis upon which acupuncture was

established. Homeopathy believes in the existence of Vital Energy; in fact, it is a primary requirement for a homeopath or a "holistic" physician. Western medicine tends to overemphasize the analytical side, as if the human body could be broken down into a definite set of facts and drawers. By reducing the body to *Gray's Anatomy,* modern medicine fails to see that Vital Energy has no material existence and, therefore, cannot be dissected like other parts of the body.

3. Health is harmony of vital processes. Disease has its beginnings in the disturbance of this harmony: this is the fundamental law of homeopathy. In modern terms, disease begins in some imbalance of electromagnetic processes, which precipitates a change in body chemistry; this change, if not reversed, results in tissue changes, called pathology--the end result of disease. Traditional medicine regards pathology as the disease itself and seeks to remove it, thinking, thereby, that they are curing the patient. This folly continues today.

4. Diseases are consequences of a disturbed Vital Energy, and as such are <u>effects</u>, not causes. Illnesses are the result of exposure to harmful influences: emotional, mental, and physical. If these pernicious triggers are stronger than the present Vital Energy in the person, then disorder or discomfort (dis-ease) will follow. What is worse, Western medicine breeds disorder by introducing vaccines, drugs and invasive harmful techniques, undermining an already disturbed energy, leaving behind a greater disorder than before. This is one of the great delusions of modern medicine: *it replaces a small disorder with a greater one.* A typical example is the continued misuse of antibiotics, which are prescribed for mere colds and flus. After 50 years of abuse, medicine finally has started to recognize the harm that has been done: increased presence of yeast overgrowth; prolonging of the natural course of colds and children's

diseases; and the resurgence of TB, syphilis and gonorrhea because of resistance to existent drugs are all noted consequences.

5. Disease is a conflict between two parties: on one side, the provoking agent (microorganism); on the other side, the living subject (the patient) undergoing the aggression. The first part is all too overemphasized in Western medicine, while the second part disappears into oblivion. For any given disease, the search is on for the tiny offender but, reinforcement of the victim is advised all too rarely. Why is it that in epidemics some people get sick and others do not? This is due to *inherent causes*, a *morbid receptivity*, and a *lack of natural defense* of the individual. As long as the defense system is intact, we are resistant to most exterior aggressions. "The virus means nothing, the terrain is everything." It is time that allopathic medicine starts paying attention to the recipient instead of the aggressor only.

6. Health is the balanced state of the body and mind in an individual. The Vital Energy controls the harmony between body and mind. This normal health and the harmonious Vital Energy depend on Hygiene (nutrition, ventilation, personal and social hygiene, water supply) AND absence of a hereditary disease dyscrasia or miasma. Otherwise, the psychosomatic makeup of the individual is abnormal from the beginning. Homeopathy can successfully prevent the onset of many chronic diseases by regulation of hygienic measures and constitutional treatment of the present miasma. True jewels of internal Hygiene are: diet, Tai Chi, Qigong, meditation, mental hygiene and lucid dreaming.

7. From paragraph 6, it is evident that a homeopathic remedy by itself will not be successful if Hygiene has not been taken

into consideration. Hahnemann states in Paragraph 77 of the Organon:

" Those diseases are inappropriately named chronic which persons incur who expose themselves continually to avoidable noxious influences, who are in the habit of indulging in injurious liquors or aliments, who reside in unhealthy localities, who are deprived of exercise in open air, who live in a constant state of worry, etc............"

It seems to me that Hahnemann is correctly describing the sorrowful present situation. It is imperative for the physician, before prescribing the appropriate homeopathic remedy, to discuss all the possible blocks on the road to recovery. All too often, the patient expects nothing short of a miracle from the remedy (much greater is the expectancy of the patient and much shorter his patience than is the case after the prescription of a regular drug), without feeling the need to change his life-style. Nothing less is true. Before the physician changes a well-prescribed remedy, he needs to discuss roadblocks on the way to health again on the second visit (see "Obstacles to the Cure," page 58). Otherwise, he might feel compelled to change inappropriately the prescribed remedy, with disastrous consequences: the case becomes incurable.

8. *"Therefore disease (that does not come within the province of manual surgery) considered, as it is by the allopathists, as a thing separate from the living whole, from the organism and its animating vital force, and hidden in the interior, is an absurdity, that could only be imagined by mind of materialistic stamp, and for thousands of years given to the prevailing system of medicine all those pernicious impulses that have made it a truly non healing art."* Paragraph 13, Organon, 6th Ed.

What a condemnation of "modern" medicine by Hahnemann in his time. Alas, not much has changed in 200 years. Most modern physicians still practice as if the body and mind are two separate entities. The doctor looks for any subtle anatomical and laboratory change, while the psychiatrist or psychotherapist seem to feel that a human being is only composed of the mind. Therefore, a psychotherapist, not knowing the physical symptoms of the diseased state, will declare the patient "healed" after dwelling long enough on the past. My only hope is that one day homeopathy will be part of the psychotherapist's curriculum. Results would be achieved in less than half the time, and by obeying and recognizing the laws of homeopathy, a true cure would be effected.

9. The true physician approaches the diseased person from a viewpoint which includes all three levels of human expression: *mental, emotional and physical.* All of them have an influence on the Vital Energy and need to be elaborated on in taking a patient history. This is, of course, true for any chronic disease. Only in this manner can the true cause or beginning of the disease be discovered and remedied. How can we cure the end product of a disease if we don't understand the beginnings? It speaks for itself, that if the patient comes to visit with an acute problem (sore throat, sprained ankle, etc.), there is no need to delve into the patient's past at first. He wants immediate relief from the discomfort. Later however, appropriately prescribing a constitutional remedy can avoid recurrence of the problem.

10. "*Nature heals while the physician amuses the patient.*" I wish modern medicine would keep this more in mind. In many instances, the Vital Energy is strong enough to overcome many acute situations with the aid of some hygienic measures, well-known by our grandmothers (rest,

warm drinks, more sleep...). In general, acute illnesses which are not serious will almost always cure themselves. Thus, about 50% require nothing but *Sac. lac.* Western medicine often slows down the natural course of disease with unsuitable drugs (see "Suppression").

Recently, a Western medical study showed a prolonging of the course of childhood diseases after administration of fever-suppressing drugs such as Tylenol™ and aspirin. Homeopathy, because it follows the laws of true healing, will stimulate the direction of the cure, without suppressing the Vital Energy. Often I have seen my patients recover from a flu in two days, while their friends, after taking several kinds of antibiotics, are still sick from the same flu after three weeks. What a loss of energy, finances and, especially, what a loss of Vital Energy! Don't forget: "*Medicines do not cure. Nature does. Do not interfere with Nature.*"

11. Homeopathy has not finished its task until the Vital Energy is restored. The Qi is in balance when the following signs of health have been obtained: refreshed sleep, adaptability to change, a sense of well-being, clarity of mind, a sense of humor, calmness, a good appetite, humility and love for life. These factors are discussed more extensively in my book *"Human Condition: Critical."*

12. When a man is happy in his surroundings, his work and his habitat, one seldom finds recurring ill health, no matter how damp and miserable the climate. This explains why physicians and nurses tending to people in the midst of an epidemic don't get sick. They are too busy working and enjoying what they are doing.

13. Homeopathy is concerned mainly with therapeutics, whereas Western medicine is concerned mainly with

diagnostics. The object of homeopathy is to raise therapeutics from its all-time condition of an empirical art to that of an art guided by laws and principles. By "proving" the remedy, which is noting the effects of remedies on healthy subjects, homeopathy teaches how to differentiate remedies to suit individual cases. To bring about a cure, we must enhance the curative process that is already occurring within the patient. The beauty of homeopathy lies in its depth; its danger arises from its shallow application by unscrupulous practitioners calling themselves "homeopaths."

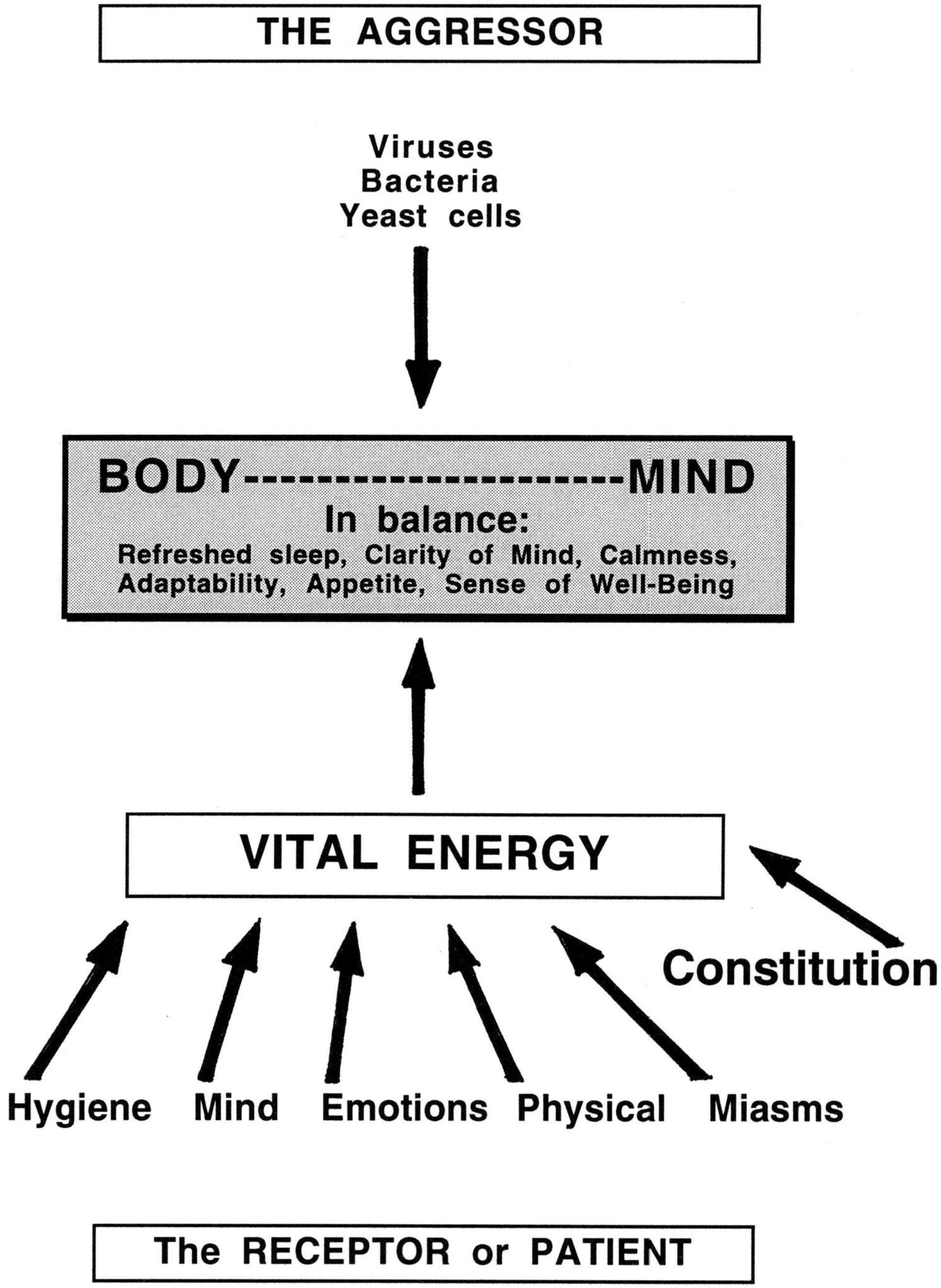
THE AGGRESSOR
Viruses
Bacteria
Yeast cells
BODY--------------------MIND
In balance:
Refreshed sleep, Clarity of Mind, Calmness,
Adaptability, Appetite, Sense of Well-Being
VITAL ENERGY
Constitution
Hygiene
Mind
Emotions
Physical
Miasms
The RECEPTOR or PATIENT

HOMEOPATHIC PRINCIPLES AND LAWS

14. A specialist, to do the most good for his patient, must be a homeopath first and then a specialist; not a specialist first and then select remedies <u>locally</u>, according to the homeopathic relations to the local part. Homeopathy holds, first of all and before everything else, a consideration of the patient as a unit, even before consideration of any of the parts.

15. You are not treating a disease but a <u>person with the disease</u>. This is an essential difference with Western medicine. Modern medicine prescribes for the patient's disease, not for the patient. One of the major goals of present medicine is to name or catalog each disease. Once this is done, the next step is a "standard" treatment, identical for each patient suffering from that disease. What an irony! This is the major reason why there are so many "incurable" diseases. Take CFIDS, for example. Much money and time is spent in search of that "guilty" elusive virus. As usual, Western medicine puts the cart before the horse. For instance, take three victims of CFIDS: One person has never been well since experiencing a heartbreak, the second one since taking the birth control pill, and the third since undergoing an operation. Yet the end result is the same--they all have the same CFIDS symptoms. So how could we think, looking at the different triggering factors, that there must be one virus causing this condition and that these three people need the same treatment. How ridiculous! In homeopathy, thy would be treated with different homeopathic remedies, aimed at the triggering factor or onset of the disease, as common sense dictates.

16. Homeopathy does not need a name for a disease. It looks at the person as a whole and tries to find contributing factors that decreased the Vital Energy. It is more than copying formulas and prescriptions from lecture notes. It requires meticulous study of each patient. This effort, this concentration and study of the action of medicine on the healthy as well as on the sick, entails constant application. Many times, your patients will ask: "Do you have a remedy for tinnitus, for back pain, for vertigo, for arthritis, etc. Your answer must be: We have a remedy for a person with tinnitus, back pain, vertigo, arthritis, etc.

17. To the true homeopath (I should say physicians in general), a cure consists of but one thing, and that is the ***eradication*** of the predisposition to the disease to be cured. A remedy does not apply a palliative action which merely deadens the pain somewhat for 15 minutes or so, only to return even more severely and with additional, even more annoying symptoms. The homeopath implies a medicinal agent entirely compatible with the malady, which completely eradicates the pain in the course of a few hours, so that it does not recur again for a long time, possibly the rest of the patient's life. The cured patient feels better (has a sense of well-being), appears healthier to those close to him (who often remark how well the patient looks and ask, "What have you been doing? You look so good"), the pathological conditions are eliminated, and he is less susceptible to the development of acute or chronic disease.

18. This type of healing is almost never achieved in Western medicine. Let's take two common examples: recurrent ear infections in children are the curse of our times, "necessitating" repeated intake of heavy-duty antibiotics. What happens? The physician continues to prescribe these drugs, which in the long run lead to other diseases, such as yeast

overgrowth with its multiple symptoms. It doesn't occur to him that he is contributing to disorder in an already weak and fragile human being. But if you ask him to do something to prevent the recurrence of this illness, he will shrug his shoulders. Should this physician really take pride in his achievements? Of course not. His allopathic treatments contribute more than their share to the decline of the human species. The second example is the perpetual vaginal yeast infection. Women are subjected to the abuse of the physician who continues to prescribe creams and drugs which suppress symptoms but never cure them. What the physician sees as a cure is in this case, really a dissipation of life energy, weakening the patient and keeping her on the road to impaired health. Patients will have to turn to a science like homeopathy to achieve a cure for these maladies.

19. *"Nature never leaps in jumps; it always goes slow."* This is probably the hardest lesson to learn for every patient and physician alike who have become used to the sudden, jerky action of Western drugs. You take a sleeping pill and you will fall asleep in a half hour. Take this anti-anxiety pill and you will feel better in 10 minutes. But is anything achieved except lulling the patient into the false belief that a "cure" has been obtained? Patients will come to you, the alternative physician, and tell you: "I will give you a month to cure my illness" (which has been present for the last 20 years!) Do you think they would say something like that to their regular physician? Never. It will take a lot of persuasiveness to convince your patient that the destruction of the Vital Energy took 20 years, and that it will take more than a month, a remedy and some praying to get well. It will take commitment to a new life-style, recognition of past errors, and time--yes, time to restore the Vital Energy.

20. Common sense dictates that one cannot kill the root of the tree by merely chopping off its individual branches, any more than one can remove the cause of a disease by removing only certain of its peculiar symptoms. Yet common sense is rarely practiced by physicians and other health practitioners, "holistic" or not. The increased specialization has favored this course. You have a sore shoulder and it is as if your shoulder comes for a consultation, not your whole person. A group of symptoms, which we so inadequately call "syndrome" (our whole tree), is chopped into individual symptoms (our branches) and given disease names to be treated, such as fibromyositis, PMS, TMJ, depression, anxiety, mitral valve prolapse (MVP), interstitial cystitis, etc.. No wonder the patient does the tour of specialists. Each of these specialists will concentrate on what he recognizes in the syndrome and treat it forcefully, distorting the whole picture even more. A cure is <u>never</u> achieved in these cases.

21. What is the cause of disease? If we have to name one common denominator, the basic cause of all disease can be summed up in a single term--<u>shock</u>. The inciting causes may be mental, physical, chemical or mechanical but if they cannot produce shock, there will be no disease. Shock simply breaks the lines of communication between the central organization of the body and the traumatized part involved.

22. Experience has a place in science, but only a confirmatory place. It can only confirm that which has been discovered through principle, or law, guiding us in the proper direction. Experience does not lead to discoveries. One who has no doctrines, no truth, no law, who does not rely upon law for everything, imagines he discovers by experience. Out of his experience, he will undertake to invent, and his invention runs in every conceivable direction. This paragraph leads us to the only real question: "*On what laws and principles is a*

so-called science like Western medicine based?" On ***none!*** In other words, our only guiding lines are "hit and miss"! We have no healing principles in modern medicine guiding us in our treatment plan. So-called double-blind studies (in reality, this means twice blind, the doctor and the patient) are performed on animals and sick people whose Vital Energy is already disturbed. Western medicine is still based on *"The Contrary Kills the Contrary"* basis of the well-known germ theory.

Have you ever thought why what we were doing in Western medicine 20 years ago has almost vanished today? Proponents of this science call it progress. In reality, it was one of the many "hit and misses." So inconstant and variable is allopathy that, should an allopathic doctor die today and come back to life fifty years from now and attempt to continue his profession, he would have to graduate all over again. Not so for a homeopath, who could come back two hundred years from now and be very proficient. The only thing he hopefully would have to learn more about are new proven remedies, an extension of our Materia Medica. The only facet of modern medicine that sticks around and is considered the pride of preventive medicine is the vaccination. And guess what...it is based on the homeopathic law *"Like Cures Like."* But our allopathic friends use doses too large with far too frequent repetition, and, therefore, vaccination has disappointed more than it should have.

23. But what about *"Contraria Contrariis Curantur,"* or "the Opposite Cures the Opposite," which is almost always practiced, conciously or not, by allopathic practitioners? Purgatives are given for constipation, antipyretics for fever, pain killers for pain, sleeping pills for insomnia, etc. This could be an excellent way of practicing were it not going directly against Nature's law that *"To every action there is an*

equal and opposite reaction." The reaction to a purgative will be more constipation, to a painkiller, more pain, and so on. The result is that these drugs require ever-increasing doses, and instead of curing a disease, a drug-induced disease is added to the misery of the patient. The much-heralded principle, or fallible rule, "Contraria Contrarii Curantur," is applicable only to physiological conditions, not pathological ones. Hunger and thirst are physiological states, not diseases, and are appeased by eating and drinking. But a stroke, a rash, a boil have no contraries. Their cure can only be accelerated by helping Nature in the same direction Nature combats them, but not by interfering in the opposite direction!

24. It is time for us to look at a true scientific healing method like homeopathy and see on what laws it bases itself. We are using the word "law" and not "rule." Laws are made by infallible Nature, rules by fallible man. First, there is the law of *"Like Cures Like."* This was not necessarily Hahnemann's brainchild. Hippocrates himself understood that a sick person could not be considered apart from his environment and that illness is a condition of the whole person. In Paragraph 61 of the *Organon*, Hahnemann wrote 200 years ago:

"Had physicians been capable of reflecting on the sad results of the antagonistic employment of medicines, they had long since discovered the grand truth, THAT THE TRUE RADICAL HEALING ART MUST BE FOUND IN THE EXACT OPPOSITE OF SUCH AN ANTIPATHIC TREATMENT OF THE SYMPTOMS OF DISEASE." (Capital letters added for emphasis by author)

Hahnemann came by this conclusion from firsthand experience. At age 35, while translating a medical book, he was struck by the conflicting reports about quinine. He decided, as a true and inquiring physician, to try it on himself. After several days of administration, he began to experience the fever symptoms similar to those for which quinine was the remedy. Soon after, he experimented with other substances and came to the same conclusion: a substance can cure what it induces, or, like can cure like.

The question arises: how many physicians are willing, as Hahnemann did, to try these untested, "heroic" medicines they give to sick people on themselves? Have you looked at the quality of life of "treated" or "practiced on" patients with "incurable" diseases?

25. The use of a *single remedy* is a **second** guideline for the homeopathic physician. When the doctor decides upon a homeopathic remedy according to the totality of the symptoms (i.e., taking into account the whole person, including the emotions as well as physical symptoms), he will prescribe ONE remedy at a time. By administering this remedy by itself, the practitioner will be able to distinguish its actions from the interfering effects of other substances. Patients should not take "mixed" preparations of homeopathics, so common on the market today. Practitioners using these mixtures are not homeopaths, but just lazy--unwilling to spend the necessary years studying. Hahnemann would have nothing but contempt for these practitioners, who have the audacity to call themselves "classical" homeopaths. Hahnemann himself said,

" It is impossible from any knowledge we possess of the separate actions of remedies, to predict what will be their effects in combination."

26. As you can see, the mixing of homeopathic medicines is not only contrary to the fundamental idea of homeopathy, but it

does not allow us *a posteriori* to obtain knowledge about the actions of our medicines. If pharmaceutical companies want to develop mixtures, they should do so according to the principles of homeopathy and test their pure effects on healthy individuals (provings). Otherwise, the mixture practice is a dangerous innovation, because we don't have the slightest evidence to show that the action of a chemical compound will be at all similar to that of each of the simple substances of which it is composed. To demonstrate my point even further, in Paragraph 273 of the *Organon*, Hahnemann says:

"In no case under treatment is it necessary and therefore not permissible to administer to a patient more than one single, simple medicinal substance at one time. It is absolutely not allowed in homeopathy, the one true, simple and natural art of healing, to give the patient at one time two different medicinal substances..."

27. It is unnecessary to apply a multiplicity of means where simplicity will accomplish the end. Too many remedies administered in a single prescription confuse the vital force, neutralize the remedial effects, disorder the state of sickness, make obscure the true picture of disease, teach the physician nothing, create within his mind a spirit of infidelity in medicine, cultivate a slovenly habit of prescribing and bring discredit upon the profession of homeopathy.

28. The last thing we want to do is imitate Western medicine, in which remedies, themselves productive of disease, are given in a cumulative manner, so that the original symptoms are lost in the crowd of artificial maladies. Allopathy, by its blind routine, by its large doses of active drugs and by its complex, multiple prescriptions, is, therefore, not only ineffectual as a curative system but becomes the fruitful agent of a host of

diseases. We all know the stories of patients who come to us taking ten different drugs: five for five different symptoms; the other five to annihilate the accepted side-effects (euphemism for poison) of the first five drugs.

29. Experimentation on healthy individuals (called *Proving*) is a **third** principle and a must for any science! From ancient times until well into the 18th century, much of what was known about drugs was based on pure speculation or from the picture of poisonings. In 1666, a dean of the Paris Faculty of Medicine, Dr. Patin, wrote:

> *"They say that poison is not a poison in the hands of a good doctor. Most of them have killed their wives, their children, or their friends, and yet notwithstanding they go on to speak of a drug they themselves would not dare to touch."*

It would be helpful, even today, when many experimental drugs and vaccinations are tried on desperate people, for doctors to try these on themselves first. This is where Hahnemann's approach was revolutionary. For the first time in the history of medicine, a doctor conceived the idea of testing medicines on himself. And later, under his supervision, his pupils, mostly physicians and family members, experimented with a vast number of substances, noting all the effects. Before Hahnemann did this, the effects of drugs were only known as a result of accidental poisoning.

30. Our first question is, Who should prove drugs?
Anyone in a reasonable state of health, able to observe in himself any changes that may take place which are different from his ordinary feelings and sensations, is able to prove a medicine. A finished proving should be made by at least 50 people, including all ages and both sexes, so that the positive indicators of that particular drug can be sifted out and the

rest discarded. To be prepared for the task, the prover should note his daily state of health for a week before he begins his provings. He will then find it much easier to describe sensations and feelings that deviate from the normal. Hahnemann, in his time, proved about 100 remedies on himself without any negative effect. Such provings are not pushed to pathology, only to delicate, temporary functional or physiological symptoms. Having proved his observations in such a personal manner, it was an easy task for Hahnemann to make the observation in others.

31. What about the drug to be proved? We should always try to procure the drug or other matter in its purest state. Explain in detail how and where it was obtained and how it was prepared. Plants should be collected at the optimal time, in their original soil. If the drug is taken from an animal, it should be preserved and subsequent supplies can come from the same species. The few drops of poison taken from the Bushmaster snake by Dr. Hering, in Surinam over 150 years ago has sufficed, so far, to satisfy all the demand for Lachesis. Preparations taken from a snake while confined in a cage cannot reasonably be expected to have the same medicinal power as those from the wild snake brought alive to Dr. Hering by the Indians from the country where it was caught. In similar fashion, don't prepare remedies from plants grown in greenhouses; rather, find out where they grow wild.

32. What is the correct dose ? Hahnemann tells us in Paragraph 128 of his *Organon* to use a few pellets of the 30th potency. That does not mean that other potencies, ranging from the tincture to 1M, cannot be used. And, indeed, they have been used in provings. However, to avoid unnecessary aggravations, 30C can be applied safely. If there is no effect in the prover after, say, five days, we will have to proceed in a fashion similar to when we administer medicines for the

cure of patients: alter the potency; if no effects follow this, we can make the remedy still stronger by putting it in water. It speaks for itself that hypersensitives will be a rich source for provings. They will react faster and with a broader range of symptoms. (More about hypersensitives and their dosages under "Potencies," page 29).

33. What about regimen during the proving? The prover should continue his usual diet and habits, in general, as a deviation from them would necessarily cause some changes in his condition, and these might erroneously be considered effects of the drugs he proves. It is wise to choose provers who do not use drugs, drink coffee or tea or who usually use heavy perfume, since they might interfere with the action of the drug or even cancel it.

34. Homeopathy uses the *infinitesimal* dose: this is the **fourth** rule. Hahnemann understood perfectly well that heavy doses of a remedy would add unnecessary strain to the patient's body, which was already supporting its sickness. In order to obtain strong physiological responses from their drugs, allopaths often increase the dosage of medications, producing uncomfortable and unnatural reactions. This does not happen when the same drugs are administered in highly diluted, or homeopathic, form. There are no toxic side effects, and, since the amount of therapeutic substance is minimal, no residue is left in the body. And, of course, the clinical effects are better, as is so well-demonstrated by the 200 years of clinical research begun by Hahnemann. The minimum effective dose of the correctly chosen homeopathic remedy is always curative, pleasant and harmless.

35. Most of us have forgotten the ARNDT-SCHULTZ biochemical law, which establishes that "*Minimum doses of a drug stimulate, medium doses inhibit, higher doses destroy cellular*

activity." That homeopathic remedies can act in such small quantities is easily understood according to the concept of this law, which considered drugs as irritants. Hahnemann showed clearly that much smaller doses of the drug are needed to bring about a reaction in the diseased than in the well body, and furthermore, that in the former--especially the chronically ill--the diseased part of the body reacts much more intensely than the remaining portion.

36. If we believed that medicine would cure our patients, we might think that the more of the appropriate medicine we could administer, the quicker would be the cure, whereas exactly the opposite is true. The patient must cure himself. Medicine does not cure them. All that medicine does is *stimulate their curative powers.*

37. A contemporary of Doctor Hahnemann, CONSTANTIN HERING, M.D., a German also, wrote in 1845, two years after Hahnemann's death, his "*Guiding symptoms*" or as they are better known, ***"Hering's Laws."*** According to Hering's Laws, the disease heals and the symptoms appear:

- ❑ **From above to below**
- ❑ **From the interior to the exterior**
- ❑ **In reverse order of their arrival**

In practice, I have most often observed the validity of the second and third statements. Under the strength of the well-chosen remedy, rashes appear, discharges occur, itching becomes prevalent; in other words, the remedy helps the natural course of healing: the disease is chased <u>out</u> of the body. Discharges may temporarily increase, and yet the patient feels better. Another example of this rule: an asthma patient starts breathing better, but now he exhibits more joint pains. The disease went from an internal organ to a safer, less important part of the body, the joints. The homeopathic physician should explain this to the patient on the first visit, or, inevitably, the patient will do what he was taught by allopaths--suppress the disease with ointments. (More is discussed under "Suppression, page 80)

38. Another frightening event for the patient, if unexplained, is the reversal of symptoms in the order of their appearance. In other words, the last symptoms to appear are the first ones to disappear. If a patient comes to you and declares, "Doctor, the symptom I originally complained to you about has improved, but now I have a symptom I have not had for two years," then praise the Lord, you are on your way to curing the patient. Knowledge of these Hering's Laws by the patient and the doctor will bring understanding rather than confusion. Do not alter the remedy at this point, as the same remedy will resolve the patient's problems.

39. As a physician, we must know the difference between a *cure* and a *recovery.* Many physicians take credit for "curing" their patient, when in actuality spontaneous recovery has occurred. This is not a cure, but is related to a rallying of the Vital Energy when exiting and maintaining causes are removed. This is especially true in the case of acute diseases, where it is sufficient to rest, eat nutritiously and take extra vitamins. If the trigger was not intense, the Vital Energy will easily overcome the present obstacles. But we can't expect recovery in true chronic diseases (not to consider "chronic" because of bad habits which are maintaining causes) and recovery will not protect the patient from recurrence. In the latter case, either a constitutional remedy or removal of the miasma will be necessary.

40. A cure is quite different. In Paragraph 1 of the *Organon*, Hahnemann states:

> *"The physician's high and only mission is to restore the sick to health, to cure, as it is termed."*

There is a world of difference between restoration of health and spontaneous return to health or recovery. There will never be restoration of health without the administration of an appropriate homeopathic remedy. It is this remedy that will reactivate the Vital Energy by producing our drug (remedy) picture (which is called primary reaction), and in a second action (secondary reaction), the roused Vital Energy will remove the disease process. Recovery is achieved with the help of common sense (removal of maintaining causes) and Nature (Vital Energy). Restoration is the result of hard work on the part of the homeopath who has been able to find the simillimum, i.e., a remedy similar to the clinical picture of the patient. The cure is based on well-established homeopathic principles, with a similar logical explanation for everyone.

41. A last, but very important principle, already alluded to but too important not to repeat, is *individualization*, the **fifth** principle. The individuality of a person constitutes his distinction from others. The old saying is that "there are no two persons that look just alike." It is true not only in human beings, but likewise in all growing and living things in the animal, vegetable and mineral kingdoms. While this seems to be common sense, most physicians act as if they never heard about it. Diabetes is diabetes for them, so everyone gets treated the same way. But when we look carefully, then we see that not all these patients show the same symptoms. A homeopath will identify his patient in the true sense of the

word and, therefore, bring the patient off the road of incurability.

Kent expressed it eloquently: *"As long as man is capable of believing that diabetes is disease, he will be insane in medicine. His mind is only directed toward the results of disease.* If a physician's work were only a matter of observing macroscopical and microcospical manifestations to reveal the location of the disease, it would be easy to achieve close to 100 percent accuracy in our diagnosis. If it were possible to remove the gross pathology without destroying the patient and disturbing the physiology, our work would certainly be easier. But the distribution of our sympathetic and ortosympathetic nervous systems is so delicately arranged that no surgery can be done without affecting its harmony and function. We cannot put under a microscope mental, emotional and physical symptoms, which are the language of disorganized function and unnatural forces in the patient's body.

42 This does not mean that pathology does not have its role in the restoration of health. Dr. Constantin Hering stated that,

"No one can be a successful disciple of Hahnemann, who is not well versed, as Hahnemann himself was, in the learning of the medical schools; and it would be just as impossible for him to act judiciously without a knowledge of anatomy, physiology, pathology, surgery, together with chemistry and botany, as for a man, ignorant of navigation and seamanship, to carry a vessel with safety into port."

But to entirely rely on pathology and think that by knowing all its secrets the whole truth of the living being will be revealed is a folly in the greatest sense of the word, a folly, indeed, that is all too often adhered to in modern times.

Pathology **is** to be considered in prescribing, not as a sole basis, but as an important factor in the totality of the symptoms. It is however a tool, but by no means the leading element in the search for restoration of health.

Knowledge of pathology is a tool in the hands of the homeopath who can measure the depth of disease and predict the prognosis and possible incurability, in which case he will palliate with his remedies. This understanding will keep him from giving false promises to his patient. We also see that the pathology reveals the chronic disease in the patient: a tendency to polypi is a valuable symptom, indicating the presence of the sycosis miasm. To know pathology, even in cases which have abundant non-pathological symptoms, helps not only to satisfy the patient, but to determine our choice of potency. Low potencies will be used where the pathology is too great or the case is incurable, such as as in cancer, pneumonia, TB, etc. The use of high potencies, unless given to a vital person, would cause a severe aggravation from which the patient's system could not rally.

There is another class of pathology which we might call *objective* pathology, and it is very useful in prescribing: the presence of fissures, red orifices, herpes blisters, warts, skin lesions, nail changes, etc., which can often be our best means of determining the simillimum, especially in children.

POTENCIES

43. There is something you must learn very quickly as a future homeopath-- never enter into any discussion on potencies, for it is one thing on which homeopaths never agree. This topic will cause more feathers to fly and engender more ill-will than any other subject. But there must be a guideline for the student. Where does he start, who should he believe, what is the safest potency for his patient? I will outline my own process here, which will be very helpful to the beginner and advanced homeopath alike. I was lucky enough to get an early introduction to the LM potencies. More about that, however, later.

44. The first thing you need to realize is that there are different schools in homeopathy. In fact, there are two unicist schools, the Hahnemannian and the Kentian.

45. Both schools treat the patient according to homeopathic principles and can, therefore, be called "classical." There is only one difference. The Kentians prescribe a high potency and don't repeat until the clinical picture dictates it, often weeks or months later. This is based on the **5th** edition of the *Organon*, and was advocated and well-spread by Dr. James Kent of Chicago, a contemporary of Hahnemann. The only problem with this is that Kent never knew about the 6th edition, since it appeared after his death in 1916. Dr. Kent had, and still has, an enormous influence on homeopathic prescribing. So most classical homeopaths, with their high potency prescribing, are practicing according to the 5th edition, not the 6th. However, in his last edition (the 6th), Hahnemann rejected "everything" he had written in the 5th

edition and told his followers he had now *"found his most perfect method*," or the LM method. In fact, the last 12 years of his life were dedicated to perfecting this method. In Paragraph 246 of the *Organon*, Hahnemann states:

"What I said in the 5th edition of the Organon, in order to prevent these undesirable reactions of the vital energy, was all that the experience I then had justified. But during the last four or five years, however, all these difficulties are wholly solved by my new and altered but perfected method. The same carefully selected medicine may now be given daily and for months, ***if necessary,*** *in this way, namely after the lower degree of potency has been used for one or two weeks in the treatment of chronic diseases, advance is made in the same way to higher degrees."*

A prime example of a Kentian is the Greek homeopath Vithoulkas.

46. The Hahnemannian gives one remedy in low potency and repeats it every day (especially LM). This was totally new for homeopaths practicing according to the 5th edition. In the 5th edition, Hahnemann writes "*never to repeat the dose until there is no effect of the remedy left and symptoms are coming back after initial improvement*." The pure Hahnemannian will repeat if there is improvement, and even if there is aggravation, although only after adjusting the dose (see further). Eizayaga, an Argentine-born physician, uses 6C potencies, repeated daily, but, curiously enough, not the LM methods. In other words, he basically follows the 6th edition, although not entirely.

47. The nice thing about all of this, is that these schools can all produce results, because they adhere to the strict homeopathic rules. Please note that I never discuss giving two

different homeopathic remedies at the same time or the mixtures, which are so popular for the wrong reasons. The latter is not classical homeopathy; it is not homeopathy at all. Kentian homeopathy works best if the symptoms and problems are *functional,* Hahnemannian homeopathy works better for the more *organic* lesion. It is aimed at the disease: the diabetes, the heart disease, the arthritis, cancer, etc. So, in general, the more psychic the disturbance, the higher the potency needed. For organic pathology, prescribe low. For localized problems and skin eruptions, the potency should be low also.

48. It is common to find that the indicated remedy in chronic cases will produce excellent results in one potency but absolutely nothing in another potency. This leads to an important rule in the practice: "If a well-chosen remedy fails to work if given in low potency, it might often succeed if given in high potency." So, if you are sure of your remedy but it did not alter the clinical picture, before changing the remedy, change the potency! It will amaze the practitioner and patient alike that the same remedy in a different potency is able to eradicate all the symptoms. What a pity it would have been to abandon the remedy and possibly cause an aggravation of the illness or make it incurable. (More about this in "Management of the Patient," page 86).

49. What are the advantages and disadvantages of these different potencies? Let's start with the Kentian method. For them, high potency starts at 200C, going to 1M, 10M, etc. It is easy for the practitioner. He sends the patient home with a single dose of one remedy or gives it on the spot. Compliance is 100%, no mistakes are made. He warns the patient about the most likely aggravations and tells the patient to check back with him in another month or so. That means fewer phone calls for the physician. If the patient phones because

of an aggravation, all he has to say is, "I told you so; you have to weather the storm; phone me in one month."

50. However, disadvantages can be numerous. First, there is almost always present occurrence of an aggravation. "This is excellent," these homeopaths will say, "because it shows we selected the right remedy, since it is a similar homeopathic aggravation, i.e., the existing symptoms occur in a higher intensity." However, although an immediate aggravation after the administration of the remedy, frequently occurs, even with low potencies, there is a great difference in **intensity** of the aggravation. With high potencies, the aggravation can land the patient in a hospital (and you could lose your patient forever to homeopathy), and the aggravation can last for up to a month or more! With low potencies, this aggravation will rarely surpass two days if the remedy intake is stopped the moment the aggravation appears. This is especially true for the hypersensitives. Kentians show contempt for their patients if they do not individualize, in other words, if they don't take into account that patients will react differently to the same high potency. This is, after all, one of the basic principles of homeopathy! And Hahnemann said in Paragraph 2 of the *Organon*:

The highest ideal of cure is rapid, ***gentle*** *and permanent restoration of health,...*

Unless the practitioner deliberately experienced aggravation (maybe by doing a proving), he should not send his patients into a storm without considering the consequences.

51. There is another problem with Kentians. Because they are so afraid that this one time, one dose will be canceled by external circumstances such as camphor, mint, other medications, coffee, etc., they absolutely forbid the patient to

use any of the above. They are so rigid in their rules that they unnecesarily lose a lot of patients at the onset. Take a patient with rheumatoid arthritis or asthma, for instance. Very often these people are on high doses of steroids or other medications. Kentians refuse to treat these patients until they stop all medications. This is often impossible and if it is, often lands the patient in the hospital with an acute attack. So much for compassion.

Some Kentians that I know go even further and forbid the patient to take acupuncture treatments. This is ridiculous as acupuncture uses the same laws, and the integration of two powerful, energetic medicines is beneficial to the patient, not harmful. The intake of concentrated vitamin supplements, although not always contraindicated, often can increase the energy of the patient and cover up symptoms that would otherwise spontaneously develop. Therefore, in constitutional treatment, they are not recommended, and after a cure they are not needed if the patient is on a proper diet.

52. In reality, no matter how paranoid Kentian prescribers are in telling patients to avoid mint, coffee, and other medications or treatment modalities, these interfering factors are rarely severe enough to stop the action of the *correct* remedy. If anything interferes with the action of the remedy, it is obvious in its *intensity* and, if possible, should be removed. If patients can't stop drinking coffee immediately, let them take the remedy *after* the intake of coffee, not before, as there is much less chance that the remedy will be canceled.

53. <u>Low potency</u> prescribing has more advantages than disadvantages. By low potencies, we mean LM and 6C. Disadvantages are that you have to instruct your patient thoroughly, preferably giving him written instructions, but even then patients err in taking doses. Often I have seen the

patient take the whole cup of the LM instead of one teaspoonful. Inevitably, an aggravation follows, usually of short duration however. Since the remedy needs to be repeated daily, compliance can be a problem. It is less so with LM since there is only ONE daily dose. 6C usually requires two or three doses. Of course, phone calls to the practitioner will be more frequent. After all, you are the expert, and powerful potencies such as LM can act swiftly and sometimes need quick adjustment (see "Management of the Patient," page 85). But the excellent results you achieve make up for the extra work.

54. The advantages of prescribing LM are numerous. As I mentioned in Paragraph 53, only one daily dose is necessary, so compliance is very good. The greatest advantage is that you can adjust the dose on a daily basis as the patient starts to react to the remedy. Once the patient reacts to the first dose, the next step might be an adjustment, depending on the reaction (see "Management of the Patient," Reaction After the First Dose, page 85). This is especially important with the *Hypersensitives*, a category of patients that included only about 10% of patients in Hahnemann's time, but about 30% to 40% of patients at present. None of these hypersensitives would react very well towards a high dose remedy: the prolonged, severe aggravation would cause most of them to shy away from further treatment.

55. By prescribing LM, we can adjust the dose in many ways. Normally, the practitioner can acquire LM potencies from different pharmacies. Following is the procedure to prepare a **Remedy Solution Bottle (RSB)** for the patient: fill a clean, amber bottle of about four (4) ounces with distilled water (NO tap water please). Add about 15 drops of 190-proof everclear alcohol or 15 drops of brandy. For hypersensitives,

instead of alcohol, use vegetable glycerin. Put **one** pellet from your LM tube in the RSB.

The patient **successes** the RSB from 8-12 times. A "succussion" is a striking of the RSB against the palm of your hand or against a leather book. Each succussion makes the remedy stronger. Take one teaspoon from the RSB and put it in a cup with 4 ounces of water, stir well, take **ONE** teaspoon as his daily dose and throw the rest of the water away. Repeat the same procedure every day. First succuss the RSB, take one teaspoon. out of it and put it in a cup with 4 ounces of distilled water and take one teaspoon as your daily dose. This way, due to the succussions, each dose taken is stronger than the previous one! It is like continuing to push on the gas pedal of your car to keep it moving in a smooth, gentle but sure, way, without much danger of crashing the car.

56. Hypersensitives and children should do only two succussions. Practically, since sometimes you will not know if a new patient is hypersensitive or not, every patient should succuss two times the first two days; 4 times the next two days, if no aggravation occurs; 6 times the next two days; and stay on 8 succussions until changes occur or until he finishes the bottle. If you are sure you have a hypersensitive patient in front of you (especially patients with many environmental sensitivities, who will tell you that they reacted badly to every medication they tried in the past), you should advise them to succuss two times a day while using the first bottle. (And NO alcohol in the RSB).

57. If there is an immediate aggravation after taking a dose of the LM solution, be it after the first dose or later, it signals that "our car goes too fast and crashes." We need to adjust, and this is where LM potencies have no equal. Whereas high potencies (200C, 1 M, etc.) leave the patient helpless in the

storm, with these we can adjust immediately. First, **stop** the remedy for two days. During this time period, the aggravation will disappear, as the body will use up the surplus of the remedy. The patient improves each day nothing is taken. The third day, the patient will adjust the dose. The best adjustment is doing <u>fewer successions</u>, but still taking the remedy every day. As a general rule, the patient is better off taking the remedy every day with fewer succussions, than taking the remedy less frequently with more succussions.

For example, let us say that the patient was succussing 8 times for 5 days when the aggravation occurred. After waiting two days, he will succuss 6 times every day. Often there will be no further aggravation. If there is, it is obvious that fewer succussions (5,4,3...) are indicated. Another dose adjustment is skipping the intake of the remedy, taking it every other day with the same or fewer succussions. A third method is to use more water in the RSB. Instead of a 4 ounce bottle, use an 8 ounce bottle. A final adjustment can be made by putting a teaspoon from your first cup (the patient's normal daily dose) in a second, third or more cups, and taking the daily dose from that second, third, etc., cup.

58. Never allow the patient to take more than ONE teaspoonful from the cup as the daily dose. To many patients it is hard to believe that a tiny amount of remedy (or a little water, as they call it) will result in anything. But to their surprise, when they take more of it (sometimes the whole cup by accident, or to prove to themselves that this "water" has no effect), immediate aggravation occurs and respect for the remedy is established. I have also seen practitioners fall into this trap. After choosing the proper remedy, and achieving excellent results, they give two doses daily instead of one, "to speed up the process." Often a case which has been going

well will be botched and even made irreparable (although rare with LM). Remember, in homeopathy more is not better!

59. Other advantages of prescribing LM are:

- ❑ The lowest of the LM potencies can act as deeply as the high C potencies and yet be gentle enough not to do harm in pathological cases.
- ❑ If the patient antidotes the remedy by drinking coffee for example, the daily use of the ascending potencies will quickly overcome this.
- ❑ The patient understands this method more easily because of its resemblance to the allopathic method of dosing, namely, on a daily basis.
- ❑ Because of the quick and clear action of LMs, disruption of the case by the wrong remedy is quickly noted, and also wears off much more quickly than a disruption created by high potency centesimal (C) doses.

60. Potency symbols:

- ❑ **MT.** = Mother tincture: alcohol extract of a soluble substance, not potentized. Usually stored in 100% alcohol.
- ❑ **LM** = 1:50,000 C, also written as LM/1, LM/2, 0/1, 0/2 or Q1, Q2, etc.. Our favorite potency for chronic cases, but can be used for acute cases, too.
- ❑ **X** = 1:10 (decimal scale), also written as **D** in Europe. Potencies less than 12 X (= 6C) will rarely be used. Being too close to MT., they will often aggravate.
- ❑ **C** = 1:100 (centesimal scale) also written as **CH** (Centesimal Hahnemaniann) in Europe. **6C** is the lowest commonly used centesimal potency for chronic cases--if LM is not available--or in rare cases where a patient reacts better to the centesimal potencies than the LM potencies (about 20%). **30C** is the most useful potency in acute cases and constitutional cases (although in the latter, 1M or 10M is preferable). **200C** is the most difficult potency to use.

Beginners should not try this. If it is right, it gives marvelous results. If it is wrong, it gives the worst aggravation, even worse than 1M. Many <u>nosodes</u> are in 200C potency, although nosodes may be used in other potencies, such as 6C.

- ❑ **1 M** = 1,000C; it is the easiest, safest and gentlest of all higher potencies. Good to administer after several LM potencies to progress the case faster without unnecessary aggravations. Also excellent for constitutional prescribing or in case there is an acute trauma and your patient is not sensitive. Action lasts about 3-4 weeks.
- ❑ **10 M** = 10,000 C; used for injury and operations (pre- and postoperatively); follows after 1M if the case is not resolved yet. Action lasts about 6-8 weeks. Excellent for constitutional prescribing.
- ❑ **CM** = 100,000 C; usually follows when lower potencies (1M, 10M) cease to work and the case is not resolved. Not often necessary.

61. There is a great deal of evidence to suggest that if one gets a brilliant result with a 10M, one would have achieved the same result with a LM or 6C potency, with fewer aggravations. One always has to remember that the body can become accustomed to a potency. This is what leads me to favor the course of getting as far as possible with a low potency, so that there is still a complete armory of higher potencies left when the patient no longer responds to a potency. Remember not to repeat higher potencies (from 200C on) more than 2 times. Then a higher potency is required for further action (200C-200C-1M-1M-10M-10M-50M-50M-CM-CM-MM-MM). If we have gradually reached the highest potency and there is no further response, it has been found, in such cases, that susceptibility to the remedy in the lower range is often restored. It is customary to start with the 30th potency again.

62. You have to be able to use all potencies in homeopathy. A physician who does not use all potencies fails to get out of homeopathy all that is possible. Some other potencies prescribed by old masters in chronic cases were: 30C once a week for several weeks; or a 10M potency three times with a 12-hour difference; or 200C, one dose, and wait until repetition is needed. Dr. Pierre Schmidt from Switzerland used 30C, 200C and 1M in acute traumas, one dose from each with 4 hours interval and had remarkable speedy recoveries. The beginner should stick to the guidelines expressed in previous paragraphs.

63. As a resumé for potency selection:

High potencies	**Low potencies**
❑ No pathology	Marked pathology
❑ Mainly mental symptoms	Hypersensitives
❑ Terminal stage of disease	Miasmatic depth of illness
❑ Dying patient/euthanasia	The very aged
❑ Acute diseases	Weak patients
❑ Sluggishly-reacting patients	
❑ Acutely sick strong patients	
❑ Children, esp. for constitution	

High potencies: 200C and above. Low potencies: mainly, 6C and LM.

PRESCRIBING

64. It is only by doing your very best work that you will maintain your reputation and be able to cure the sick. Successful prescribing depends on an intense study of each individual case. Hasty prescriptions not only fail to cure, but they confuse the case by hiding the simillimum. Such prescriptions may ameliorate some of the symptoms and prevent others from manifesting themselves, thereby masking the overall picture.

65. Failure to find the simillimum prolongs the case, requiring many visits from the patient and hindering recovery. Finding the simillimum is dependent upon your knowledge of our Materia Medica. The simillimum is the ideal, but what is this "similarity"? Similar to what? To objective conditions, anatomical lesions and subjective symptoms. But clinical experience has taught us that for the purpose of homeopathic prescribing, the *characteristic* individual symptoms of the patient offer the surest similar to be met and covered by a remedy having similar characteristics. One of the great advantages of homeopathy is that it can read the *language of Nature*, i.e., the totality of the symptoms, while the disease is in the functional stage, and the homeopath can administer a remedy to prevent further illness. This is true preventive medicine. The symptoms are the sole expression of internal disturbance which nature gives us in time to effect a cure.

66. The more prominent, uncommon, peculiar and rare features of the case should be noted carefully. For these in particular should bear the closest similarity to the symptoms of the remedy. The more general and indefinite symptoms, such as lack of appetite, headache, weakness, insomnia, distress, etc.

unless more closely defined, deserve little notice because of their vagueness and because such generalities are common to every disease and to almost every remedy.

67. The situation expressed in Paragraph 66 is a common mistake of the novice. He will take a case and present his preceptor with fifty symptoms. To his amazement, the experienced preceptor will throw out all but three symptoms and match these with a remedy. It is one of the grave errors of Western medicine to forego specificity of symptoms. Rarely does a doctor go into detail to better define and distinguish from other cases symptoms such as fatigue, depression, rheumatic pains, etc. Common symptoms have no place in the selection of our remedies. In fact, *the greater the value of a symptom for diagnosis* (or should I call it name-giving?), *the less its value in the remedy selection.* No wonder allopathic medicine has such trouble finding a solution for chronic diseases and is content with breaking down the symptom-totality to little groups of symptoms, naming it fibromyositis, PMS, TMJ, depression, etc. This name-giving only hides the incompetence of the allopathic physician to view the symptom-totality and to match it with **ONE** medication, instead of the multitude of drugs fired randomly at the unsuspecting patient.

68. The *symptom-totality* consists solely of that ***small*** pathogenic direct group of symptoms that a drug alone can produce in ***every*** individual and which never varies. In other words, this remedy, proven by different people, will consistently produce the same symptoms. They are the symptoms in third degree or fat caps in our repertory. Prescribing on the *"Totality of Symptoms"* is one of the prerequisites to homeopathic prescribing. However, the totality of symptoms is not merely a numerical sum of all the symptoms indiscriminately. It means all the symptoms of the

case which are capable of being logically combined into a specific and consistent entity according to the importance of symptoms expressed in Paragraph 72.

69. But we cannot be rigid about "symptom-totality." If, for instance, Bryonia in itself directly produced all the symptoms listed in Allen's Materia Medica, then **all** those symptoms **must** be present in every case calling for Bryonia if we are to have the true picture of Bryonia. Has anyone ever used that entire list? If not, then no one has ever made a true Bryonia prescription. The truth is that the homeopath uses from the above an *essential* list of symptoms every time he prescribes Bryonia, not always in its entity, but *always* in part.

70. What are peculiar symptoms? Study of the Materia Medica allows you to recognize **keynote symptoms** of each remedy: thirstlessness with fever of Apis and Pulsatilla; desire to curse and swear of Anacardium; the clean tongue with nausea and vomiting of Ipecac; the strong desire for open air of Pulsatilla; the improvement of pain by laying on the painful side of Bryonia; the pasty white tongue of Antamonium crudum, etc. The more one knows his Materia Medica, the more alert the prescriber will be and note these peculiar symptoms spontaneously expressed by the patient.

71. The prescribed remedies must correspond to the characteristic, striking and peculiar symptoms of *both the mental and the physical.* If one prescribes on mentals only, this can be palliative, just as prescribing on local physicals can only be palliative.

72. The "value" of symptoms is often forgotten in homeopathy, or if not, is somewhat confusing, depending on who you talk to. In practice, I have found the classification of the famous

Swiss homeopath Pierre Schmidt of Geneva the most handy. The value of symptoms depends on three pillars:

- ❑ **the Nature of symptoms**
- ❑ **the Peculiarity of symptoms**
- ❑ **the Age of the symptoms**

❑ *the nature of symptoms:* in order of decreasing importance, we classify the symptoms as:

a. mental symptoms b. general symptoms c. desires and aversions d. sleep symptoms e. sexual symptoms. For further information, see "Case Taking, page 68)

❑ *the strange and peculiar symptoms:* In Paragraph 5, we commented on the importance of the natural defense of the patient. In a community of people living in similar circumstances, all the healthy and normal individuals react in a similar way. They laugh at something funny, they perspire and are thirsty when it is very hot. On the other hand, when someone laughs at something sad, or he perspires when it is cold, we can conclude that his natural defense deviates from the normal. Other peculiar symptoms are thirstlessness with fever, improvement of pain upon pressure, a time of the day or night at which the symptom always appears, thirstlessness with a dry mouth, etc.

This second category of symptoms (the first one being the symptoms caused directly by the determined cause) varies from individual to individual and is important since it will show the kinks in the patient's defense armor where the disease will enter, hook itself and become chronic. As Sherlock Holmes said, *"That which is out of the common is usually a guide rather than a hindrance."* Curing the first category of symptoms as is done in Western medicine, inevitably leads to a relapse or another disease. E.g., in cancer, we cut, burn or medicate the cancer, yet we do nothing for the recipient, the patient. The patient's energy, under the stress of our intervention, is often suppressed. Often I see that cancer patients, a couple of years after their initial treatment, relapse with a metastasis to other organs or succumb to secondary infections. As long as allopathic medicine does not strengthen the second part of disease, the human being who experienced the attack, it will fail in its mission, which is to cure the victim. Holistic medicines such as homeopathy and acupuncture, as well as strengthening techniques such as meditation, Qi Qong, Tai Chi Ch'uan and yoga, provide the key to the reinforcement of the patient. While obliterating the first category of symptoms (killing the germs) never leads to a full cure by itself, treating the individual disturbances of the natural defense is often enough to eliminate the pathological action of the microorganism.

❑ *the age of symptoms:* It is not always easy to find the initial symptom picture of the patient. By the time of the consultation, other things have happened to the patient, obscuring the original picture. However, it is very important to find the original thread, the original symptom complex, before treatment has altered the picture. "*Never well since*" (nws) is an important clue to be picked up by the homeopathic physician, no matter what the subsequent symptoms are. Much importance also has to be given to symptoms of infancy, e.g. fears and phobias, teething problems, late speech and walking, or food/environmental intolerances in the first year of life. These symptoms will be of utmost importance in determining the constitutional remedy. However, the most recent symptoms are the most significant in determining the choice of a remedy. If a patient experienced the symptoms he suffers in the order a, b, c, d, e, then they should disappear, if the cure is perfect and permanent, in the order e, d, c, b, a.

73. There are **four classes of mental symptoms**.

The most important ones are related to the WILL. The most fundamental instinct of mankind is self-preservation. Hence, the deepest aberration would be suicidal impulses and attempts. Loathing of life, complete indifference, and fears of death, darkness, misfortune, thunderstorms and animals also fall in the classification of the will.

The second group deal with the EMOTIONS. They include the loves and hates, apprehension, desire or aversion for company, weepiness, tidiness, low self-confidence and self-worth, loquacity, taciturnity and hypersensitivity (easily offended). Also included here are recurrent dreams, such as amorous dreams, dreams of the dead, accidents, etc.

The third class belongs to the INTELLECT. They include the memory, mistakes, confusions and concentration.

The fourth group are the symptoms related to the VITALITY. They include symptoms from conditions such as *"Ailments from." E.g.,* ailments from grief, anticipation, fright, anger, mortification, vexation, disappointed love, etc., as well as sexual reactions insofar as they apply to the whole person: aversion to coitus, onanism, perversions, nymphomania, etc.

74. The greatest difficulty the beginner confronts in his early attempts to discover the simillimum, after ascertaining the totality of symptoms, is that he has discovered so many remedies in his search which bear a strong resemblance to each other. It is difficult for him to understand why any one remedy of the group is not just as appropriate to his case as any of the others. All seem alike to him. The first step in finding his solution is to dismiss from his thoughts all these similar elements and find the differences of the different

drug actions. So the problem of specific prescribing is, for the most part, made up of <u>this two-fold combination of similarity and difference</u>. For instance, take the common symptom, lack of thirst with fever of Apis and Pulsatilla. Some of the mental symptoms such as the jealousy of Apis versus the gentle, easygoing nature and weepiness of Pulsatilla will guide us to the correct remedy.

75. All of us who have been in general practice recognize the value of isolating certain symptoms. "I am better at this time," or "I am worse at this time," or "I am entirely rid of my trouble if I do certain things." If we could collect the ameliorations, the aggravations, and the modalities of the various remedies as we study them, we would be better prescribers, basing our selection of remedy on the differentiating symptoms.

76. The homeopathic physician must also learn to read between the lines; as a rule, the symptoms of which the patient complains the loudest are not always the most indicative or important in selecting the simillimum. The initial examination is the most important, and the measure of success depends largely upon its exactness and scope. If the examination is inadequate, then the remedy selected must necessarily be inadequate to cure the diseased condition for which it was prescribed.

77. Those in modern medicine who insist upon pathology as a *basis* of therapeutics, who look upon the single objective symptom and its nearest organic origin as the subject for treatment, who deride the notion of prescribing based upon the totality of the symptoms, and claim to be more than symptom discoverers, in that they aim to remove the cause of the disease--these colleagues are as false in their pathology

as they are faithless to the doctrines, and impotent as to the successes of the founder of the homeopathic school.

78. The value of the homeopathic remedies cannot be measured by pathological anatomy. Natural and drug diseases are two entirely different conditions: the laws of one have no power in the other. It is for this reason that in *studying a disease, think that all remedies may help in the case; in studying a remedy, think that it may help in every disease.*

79. Other requisites for successful prescribing are knowledge of human nature and the ability to read, interpret and evaluate the make-up of a patient. This is not just a matter of intuition, but is often the fruit of carefully studying the patient from the moment he or she walks in. If you have time, go and greet your patient in the waiting room; observe their posture, their face, the way they shake your hand, etc. (For further information, see "Homeopathic Case-taking," page 68).

80. There is a trend among certain homeopaths to sneer at acute diseases. For them, these acute events are of no importance. Calling themselves constitutional prescribers, they feel that administration of the constitutional remedy will resolve everything. I don't think this shows much compassion. Every acute event, be it traumatic, emotional or viral, constitutes a leakage of energy for the patient, and therefore needs to be remedied. If a patient consults for a sprained ankle, it is preposterous for the homeopathic physician to inquire about child abuse in his past. The first and only goal, as Hahnemann expressed it so well, is "to cure gently and rapidly." The acute trauma is the most outer layer and needs to be addressed FIRST.

81. Approximately 70% of the time, people will require one constitutional remedy throughout their life. Of the 30% that change, in most instances, the correct simillimum was not ascertained in the first place. There are very few truly constitutional remedies. These are mostly substances involved in basic physiological processes, such as sulfur, calcium (Calc.Carb., Calc-p), sodium (Nat.-mur., Nat.-c), and silica. Many polychrests, such as Lycopodium, Sepia and Pulsatilla, are composed largely of these substances.

82. <u>When should we prescribe the constitutional remedy?</u> When all the layers are peeled off and we want to prevent reoccurrence of the acute stages, e.g., recurrent ear infections in children, repeatedly requiring Belladonna. To go against this tendency and really cure the patient, Calc. Carb. in a constitutional dose (1M, 10M) is required. It is important that a constitutional remedy be repeated *infrequently*, with *long intervals* between, and only when the symptoms demand it. The true constitutional remedy should be repeated only if it does not act completely or if the symptoms are unchanged after an insufficient improvement.

83. The general rules for administering and repeating a remedy are as follows:

❑ For *<u>acute cases</u>*: use the 30C of a remedy and give three pellets twice a day or, even better, put **one** pellet of the 30C in 4 ounces of water, and take little sips about every 30 minutes. This last method is especially effective in children's infections. In these acute cases, the symptoms are very violent, so the action of the remedy is rapidly overtaken by the disease, and it may be necessary to repeat frequently as we described. But as soon as improvement occurs, stop the remedy and don't give anymore until the improvement ceases or other symptoms occur which call for a remedy. Be sure to have the correct remedy the first time, as it will save time in most instances. If you give the wrong one, it can mask the case enough that it will be almost impossible to select the remedy which would have proved curative if administered at the onset

❑ For *chronic cases:*

If there is pathology, use LM potencies (one dose daily) or 6C (3 pellets twice to three times daily). If there is no pathology and you are dealing with only functional and psychological problems, then you can use Kentian potencies. Start with 200C, one dose (3 pellets), and **wait**. If the indicated remedy has not acted after 3-4 weeks, repeat it. If there is still no improvement after another 3-4 weeks, go to 1M. If the patient improves, repeat the high dose (1M) only two times; the next dose will require a higher potency (10M). Always allow a long interval between these high potency doses: your main guideline is the patient's complaints. If, after initial improvement lasting weeks to months, symptoms seem to recur, repetition will be necessary. (See more about this in "Management of the Patient," page 85).

If the case is very clear, one can give a 10M potency immediately (except in the case of very sensitive patients). For instance, for acute trauma in a healthy sports man, Arnica 1M or 10M will bring quick and lasting relief. In general, the jump from 10M to 50M, or from CM to 500M, is not a large enough potency change for satisfactory reactions. Therefore, go from 1M to 10M to CM to MM when indicated. Be aware of the fact that the LM potencies also work for non-pathological and psychological cases. It's my opinion that LM potencies are the best any time.

84. It is best to wait at least 3 days after the beginning of the menstrual period before taking a constitutional remedy. In

addition, you should not start a remedy less than one week before the menses, especially if there are menstrual symptoms in the complaints. Otherwise, the menses often will delay the action of the remedy or produce excessive aggravation.

85. In a "mute"case (a case with few symptoms), the best prescription will be only a *partial similar*, but it will be able to raise the vitality sufficiently to manifest additional symptoms, leading to the correct prescription. In addition, when there is a paucity of symptoms, certain remedies are able to clear a lot of "debris," making the clinical picture clearer and it will be easier to make the correct prescription. These remedies are: Sulphur, Nux Vomica, Thuja and Ferrum Phoshoricum.

86. Another helpful hint in treating mute cases is to inquire about the symptoms or remedies of the **parents.** The most common path of inheritance is from the mother to the son and from the father to the daughter. So, for a boy, look at the medical history of the mother. Also, important strong symptoms which occurred in childhood can be useful for making a prescription for the adult.

87. *"When the dose is too large to cure, man receives it as a sickness."* This should be a warning to Kentians, who sometimes prescribe indiscriminately high doses, no matter what the sensitivity of the patient is. Nothing is cast in stone. If Hahnemann were still alive today, I have no doubt that his genius would have produced guidelines and potencies beyond the LM, his final contribution to this world.

88. **If one is in doubt as to when to repeat the remedy, it is better to wait too long than not long enough.** This is the most important guideline for the patient and physician alike!

Often, it will take great effort to convince the patient of this most important rule. But do insist on it, because it will save you both a lot of headaches. Don't forget that most patients today are used to immediate effects from drugs, good or bad, but usually bad in the long run. However they often demand immediate relief, having no tolerance for the slightest discomfort, even when these symptoms signify improvement in their health. This insensitivity and intolerance, which has invaded all aspects of life, has contaminated medicine, too. But be firm and don't let the patient dictate his treatment plan alone. As long as you, the practitioner keeps on learning, and take a sincere interest in your patient, you are the guide in the plane whereas your patient is the pilot. But you definitely navigate!

89. As mentioned before, pathology can be important. Therefore, laboratory tests can be helpful in determining the gravity of the ailment and sometimes its nature, the potency selections and the organs involved. While I condemn allopathic medicine for relying too much on this tool, it is a tool, nevertheless. I am not going to throw out the baby with the bathwater.

90. Desires for certain foods are, in general, not very good symptoms by which to determine the remedy; *aversions* are more valuable. In today's world, it is hard to find many people who do not desire sweets at some point. If you ask children nowadays, they all desire pizza, sweets, hamburgers or French fries. This will not help you much in selecting your remedy. If they have an aversion to fatty foods or milk, that will be more helpful. There is a difference between desire and cravings. The craving is much more intense: the patient has to have it each day and will go to any extreme to get it (e.g., getting up at night to get a candy bar). Don't be fooled by the patient who says, "I don't crave sweets, chocolate, etc."

When you ask them if they eat them, they often say, "Sure, every day." It is hard to crave something when you indulge in it on a daily basis. Likewise, when the individual has been on special diets and has voluntarily restricted or increased certain foods, the desires and aversions are less helpful. Instead ask about their habits *before* they changed their diet.

91. As for the treatment of babies, if the mother is still breast-feeding and has symptoms, she should be treated rather than the baby (in order to avoid that the illness of the mother goes to the baby). If the mother is not sick, i.e., has no symptoms, or is no longer breast-feeding, then the baby should be treated directly.

92. Drugs and hormones given during pregnancy frequently result in skin symptoms in the baby. These can often be treated by Sulphur.

93. In treating periodic symptoms (every third day, premenstrually, every two weeks, every new moon, etc.) such as headaches, PMS,. etc., one should give the remedy after the latest attack has subsided. The aggravation can be intense if given before or during an attack. If the remedy is given immediately after the attack, the next one should be less intense.

94. In general, it is best to take remedies at bedtime so that they can start working while the person is resting. The next day, the patient can observe his reactions (aggravations, improvements, no change) and communicate them to his doctor. There are some exceptions to this rule. Take Phosphorus and Bellis Perennis for example. If given at night, the patient will be awake all night with a restless, hyperactive mind.

95. There are certain periods in life when the most significant symptoms emerge. This occurs especially during *pregnancy, puberty, infancy and childhood, and in the sequel of incompletely cured acute diseases.* Therefore when taking a case, pay attention to symptoms mentioned as occurring during these periods.

96. When there are many contradictions in the case, give *Sac.lac.* (sugar pellets) and have the patient return again later (2 weeks) to see which symptoms prevail. They are the ones to prescribe on.

97. When you use Kent's Repertory to find the simillimum, you must be aware that the degrees of each remedy indicate the *frequency* with which clinical cure of that symptom by that remedy has been recorded, as well as the frequency with which the symptom has been recorded in provings. They do not indicate the *intensity* of the symptoms of provers.

98. An important form of prescribing is *retrospective* prescribing. Take for example, a patient who has CFIDS symptoms. The physician prescribes the indicated remedy and it does not work. He should then give the remedy they needed at the time they had the flu that started everything (nws flu), even though they are no more flu symptoms at the time of the consultation. It is always a good idea, at the time you take the case, to write down the original symptoms and have a time-line as to how these symptoms change or disappear, or new ones appear with time. As I already mentioned, it will be one of the indicators of health, according to Hering's Law.

99. Homeopathy is very successful in *epidemic* prescribing, be it for a known illness such as measles, or an "unknown" one (according to Western medicine), since the culprit has not

been isolated, such as illnesses like CFIDS). Even where the virus is isolated, as in the epidemic of the "Four Corners," caused by the Hanta virus, modern medicine draws a blank and is virtually helpless in preventing the spread unless they are able to make a "vaccine," which is difficult and not always helpful.

How does a homeopathic physician battle and prevent the spread of an epidemic? Let's take the classic yearly flu epidemic as an example. Allopathic medicine makes a vaccine from the previously-known virus strains and prays each year that no mutation will take place. Despite possible side-effects (sometimes deaths) due to potency or dose, this gamble is taken each year with the weakest members of our society: the elderly, children and the chronically ill.

For the homeopath, it is simple. After he has seen from 10 to 20 cases, he will write down all the symptoms he found in these patients. Then he will begin sorting them out. What symptoms were present in **all** 20 victims? They are the cardinal symptoms and are used to make the selection of the remedy. At that point, if the physician has one or two remedies suited to the epidemic, it is easy for him to act prophylactically. Let's assume one child in a family of four children comes down with a flu corresponding to Gelsemium. It will be sufficient to presribe one teaspoonful of a solution in which we have put a 30C Gelsemium pellet. For several days the whole family should take a teaspoonful from the same cup as their daily dose. Cost: a cent a day, and no side effects! No one else will come down with that particular flu. Take the Hanta virus cases. All we need to do is concentrate on all the symptoms present in the victims, look for the simillimum and administer a teaspoonful to each possible victim. This is much simpler than losing time trying to isolate the virus and then still not being able to do anything. The

Beijing flu of 1993-94 responded well to Gelsemium first, then Bryonia and Kali Bichromicum. This helped people get rid of this fearsome flu strain within two to three days, while patients not getting homeopathic remedies were in bed for one to two weeks!

100. Another possible form of homeopathic prescribing is a prescription for the development of the *child in utero.* Dr. Duncan, a famous homeopath in the beginning of the century, described two cases in which women bore harelipped and cleftpalate children; one had four such children, another one eight! Duncan wondered what he could do. He went back to his embryology books and found that the abnormality occurs prior to the third month of gestation. He found it was a bone deficiency and decided it must be a lack of some of the calciums. The question was, which one? Calc. Carb., Calc.-p, Calc. Sulph.? In this particular case, the mother was very clearly a Sulphur patient, so he tried Calc. Sulph., giving it for seven months of her gestation. She bore her next child normally. He repeated this in three other cases while the baby was in utero, and the children were born normal. This opens the way for exciting new treatment ways during the early development of the child.

101. Another important consideration is the *time of conception.* Take the example of a family with four children, only one of whom has allergies. This child has experienced the same environment, diet, and family dynamics, yet is sicker then the others. There is only one conclusion: either at conception or during the pregnancy, the parent or parents were in an altered state of health. Either they were ill, took drugs, or went through emotional turmoil which decreased their Vital Energy. In this case, you should consider the mother's case first. The remedy she needed during the pregnancy indicates the remedy now needed by the child. Say, for example, that

in the fifth month of pregnancy the mother went through a separation from her husband. This heartbreak situation could call for Natrum muriaticum. The child will be born a Nat.-m. type, with all the possible symptoms of this remedy.

102. Don't forget to look into the *traumas of birth*. Was there a lack of oxygen? Any other trauma? You have to inquire about the the various age periods and scan for possible causal events. It is a cause-and-effect universe in which we live. I always tell my patients, "A disease does not occur out of the blue." There is usually a cause behind it and the search for the cause is essential to resolving the puzzle.

103. The use of *nosodes* (diseased products) can be prescribed according to the same rules which govern the prescription of other remedies. We might consider the use of nosodes in three respects: prophylaxis, acute, and chronic diseases.

❍ *prophylaxis:* Smallpox: Variolinum; Pertussis: Pertussin; diphtheria: Diphterinum; measles: morbillinum; they possibly take the place of the present vaccinations without causing any ill effects.

❍ *acute diseases*: we still prefer the use of the well-chosen remedy over the nosode, but it can be used in clearing up lingering acute illnesses. For instance, Tuberculinum in pneumonia, and Bacillinum after recurrent colds with a persistent dry cough.

❍ *chronic diseases*: the indications for the use of nosodes are:

❑ Where chronic disease immediately followed acute; this is the "never well since" (nws) situation, nws the measles, for instance.

❑ Where chronic disease was preceded by an interval of good health, prior to which repeated acute febrile illnesses occurred; e.g., Tuberculinum in a person with recurrent colds at the slightest exposure.

❑ Where it is difficult to cover the case by other remedies; apparently indicated remedies do not work, or do not hold; or where, after careful workup no remedy seems to be indicated.

❑ Where the indicated remedy has worked for some time and then stops working, in spite of dose adjustment, the nosode used as an intermediary remedy can reopen the case again. For example, if Thuja stopped working even after increasing the potency, one dose of Medorrhinum 200C should be given for two days and Thuja should start working again.

104. What about *constitutional* prescribing? Again, there can be a considerable debate among homeopaths about the use of the constitutional remedy. Some go so far as to claim that finding the constitutional remedy will resolve all the problems of the patient, no matter how many layers one finds. Constitution is the aggregate of the physical and vital powers of an individual or, put another way, his or her qualities, temperament or disposition. When is it important and when is it not important?

It is *not* important:

❑ In acute, specific, local or general diseases that separately or simultaneously attack individuals in any part or at any time and that always result from an identical morbific agent, resulting in the same symptoms in each individual. Examples: infectious-contagious diseases, traumas, transmissible diseases, parasitical diseases, etc.

❑ In acute diseases attacking several individuals simultaneously, such as epidemics.

❑ In acute diseases that simultaneously attack only a few individuals, at different times, in separate places or cities, which present the same symptoms in these few patients, resulting from the same morbific agent. Example: sporadic diseases such as "the Four Corner Disease."

❑ In acute diseases resulting from a common morbific agent such as toxic cases, venomous cases, sunstroke, avitaminosis, freezing, etc.

It *is* important:

❑ When the appropriate acute remedy cures but fails to prevent recurrence of the illness. Example: recurrent otitis media in children.

❑ At the end of the treatment of the several layers of the patient, in order to reinforce his health.

❑ In acute diseases presenting different symptoms in each patient but resulting from the same morbific agent; or in acute diseases presenting similar symptoms, but resulting from different morbific agents. Example: allergies.

OBSTACLES TO THE CURE

105. An incorrect prescription is not always due to a mistake by the doctor. One of the obstacles to be taken into consideration is laziness: the patient is too lazy to make a note of his symptoms as they occur, and when visiting the doctor, is too careless to remember his symptoms. Sometimes the patient thinks certain events are not worth mentioning.

I remember a patient telling me that the origin of her problems started when she started taking the birth control pill. I was careful and asked if there was anything else that happened to her at the onset of her illness, but she denied it. I prescribed Sepia and the only improvement we got was an improved menstrual cycle. It was clear that Sepia was not the simillimum. When I again asked about other precipitating events, she told me that at the beginning of the disease there has been a breakup with her fiance which devastated her for months, but she thought that "this was not important enough to mention," and "probably had nothing to do with my symptoms." It was a misperception by the patient. Natrum muriaticum resolved everything.

The patient's unwillingness to cooperate wholeheartedly may militate against his chances of a cure. Of course, as in the above example, post-factum, it confirmed the use of Nat-m., since they are personalities who don't like having the conversation turned to themselves; they are uncomfortable with consolation and never volunteer information. It is like pulling teeth. Very often the patient does not reveal pertinent information, considering it irrelevant or insignificant, or tries to conceal it out of a sense of shame or embarrassment. So, you often may have to take the case again.

106. One of the difficulties in homeopathic prescribing is that the American people are the most sensitized in the history of the world. They are severely debilitated by our effete way of life. For these people, any pain is intolerable and even slight discomfort must be resolved immediately. Thus the need for fast-acting drugs has been created, with an addiction plague as a consequence. Sometimes our remedies have been rendered ineffective by drugs prescribed by the most esteemed doctor of all time--the TV commercial. To reverse the effects of excessive drugging, or after excessive surgery, first prescribe Nux Vomica for two to three weeks and then choose the indicated remedy. Sometimes we can use the potentized drug that was responsible for the last layer, for example, *"nws taking Penicillin."* Penicillin 6C will nullify the ill effects of massive drugging. This is called *tautopathy.* Other antidotes are: for abuse of beer and aromatics, ***Nux Vomica***; for tea, ***Pulsatilla*** or ***Thuja;*** for quinine, ***Pulsatilla or Arsenicum***; for abuse of whiskey and hard liquor, ***Ledum***; for overindulgence in sugar, ***Argentum nitricum***; for overindulgence of fat, ***Pulsatilla*** and ***Nux Vomica***.

107. The nature of the disease--its advanced obstructive pathology is another matter of careful examination and can be an obstacle to the cure. More about this under "Palliation and Incurable Diseases," page 94.

108. Occasionally the symptoms are poorly expressed by the patient, due perhaps to lowered vitality or reduced power of reaction to the disease on the part of the patient himself. As mentioned before, studying the family history and the early childhood history of the patient can give us necessary clues, leading to the proper remedy. Sometimes we need to give a *reaction remedy* such as Sulphur, Thuja, Carbo Vegetalis, or Capsicum.

109. Another obstacle to the cure is the limited knowledge of the homeopathic Materia Medica by the professional himself. Unfortunately too many of these so-called "homeopaths" consider the study of the Materia Medica futile and a sheer waste of time. Many homeopathic pharmacies, by creating "mixtures" for a specific disease name, confirm their opinion and make it easier to give them a false sense of "good homeopathic knowledge." But mixtures, prescribed for disease names and lack of knowledge of the Materia Medica are sham-homeopathy and a disgrace to the profession.

110. The spirit of standardization, which in recent years has become increasingly manifest in the medical profession through governmental agencies and insurance companies, whose regulatory pressure continues to increase, is rapidly destroying the independence of the physician and one of the pillars of homeopathy, which is the individualization of the patient. This modern tendency may perhaps be considered the greatest obstacle to the effecting of cures by homeopathy. Insurance companies require "name giving" diagnoses: you are required to categorize them.

111. Before deciding to change your remedy, either because it is not acting or ceases to show further progress, or if the amelioration comes to a sudden halt, find out if the patient has knowingly or unknowingly interfered with the curative action of the drug. The immoderate use of alcohol, coffee, tea or marijuana can suppress susceptibility. Hahnemann's prescription regarding diet is to let the patient be the guide in acute diseases. His cravings can be judiciously gratified. In chronic diseases, the doctor will restrict them. Mere abstinence from certain foods will often remedy derangements of health when food that is too rich or too fat has been indulged in, burdening the organ, which has repeatedly sent out warning symptoms. But many are slow to recognize the danger signals, and lesions of the digestive organs soon result. The impossibility of forming rules in adhering to a diet is apparent when we find that some patients thrive on what are considered the least digestible foods, while on the other hand, some patients could not partake of any of these substances without suffering severely.

112. An obstacle easily overlooked by the physician is the presence of a miasm. In what circumstances should you suspect a miasm?

❑ If there is TB, syphillis, cancer, or gonorrhea in the history of the patient or the family, usually suppressed by modern medications.
❑ The remedies don't hold; they worked initially but have stopped working.
❑ When there is a paucity of symptoms.
❑ Return of old symptoms such as discharges, warts, polyps, rashes, etc.

The physician will have to clear the miasm before his well-chosen remedy will work again. In the course of the treatment, this may happen several times and he may feel like he is "bumping against a wall" in his treatment. His first thought should be the possibility of miasms.

113. Other obstacles are apparent. Homeopathy is a method for thinkers only, and they are in the vast minority. A more recent lull in the influence of homeopathy, and at the same time limiting its success, is the discontinuance of proving drugs, thereby causing the homeopath to to resort to allopathy to relieve what we cannot cure, since the simillimum in Nature is not yet known. This should not come as a surprise to us, since only a small percentage of the resources in nature are proved.

114. As the years go by, it seems to me that the task of homeopathic physicians is more and more difficult, the successes less direct and spectacular, and the failures more frequent. This is due to the so-called "progress" of our civilization: the ever-growing expansion of public health, with chlorination and fluoridation of our water; the drugging and alterations of our foodstuff; the air pollution by industrial fumes; the multiple vaccinations; the increasing use of X-rays; and the universal drugging with antibiotics and barbiturates. All these factors contribute to the overwhelming suppression of natural disease manifestations, which confuses and complicates the problems in selecting our remedies.

115. Everything listed under "Mistakes in Prescribing" can be considered an obstacle to the cure, though more often it is related to human failure and lack of knowledge of homeopathy.

MISTAKES IN PRESCRIBING

116. **Overemphasis of symptoms:** It is easy to pay too much attention to a single peculiar symptom and forget the totality of the symptoms. It might lead you to a rare remedy but those cases are infrequent. More important is to use the keynotes and the differentials between remedies. For each case, take these strong symptoms and you will make your case simple. You want to make sure that you find a remedy that covers the most intense symptoms. (more in "Homeopathic Case Taking," page 68).

117. **Negative matching of a remedy:** This is probably the biggest mistake in prescribing. Frequently a patient will read about his remedy in the Materia Medica and say: "I don't have this or that aspect of this remedy, so this remedy is not for me." What really counts in your prescribing is that you have at least 3 or 4 strong keynote symptoms of the remedy. This will be reason enough to apply it. For instance, you have a patient with a weepy personality, changing moods and a brooding nature, with recurrence of a thick, yellow vaginal discharge, who craves fresh air and feels better moving around. Yet the patient is very thirsty. Only the last symptom is contraindicated for the non-thirsty Pulsatilla patient, but it would be a grave mistake not to prescribe Pulsatilla in this case. Whenever you encourage your patient to read about their remedy, make sure to explain this to them: "See what matches you positively, not negatively!"

118. **Ignoring the etiology:** "Tolle causum" or "Remove the cause" is a fundamental principle emphasized by Hahnemann himself. One of the strong points of a holistic medicine such as homeopathy is that you treat the root as well as the sick

branches. Don't fall into the pitfall of Western medicine or you are practicing homeopathy in an allopathic way, which can only lead to palliation but no true cure. In fact, if the etiology is very strong, no matter what the symptoms are, the etiology will be the leader in determining your remedy. For instance, the patient has an array of symptoms (headaches, diarrhea, insomnia, vertigo, loss of memory, etc., after a head trauma. Your first choice should be Natrum Sulphuricum (with Arnica as a backup). Even symptoms that have appeared after this trauma and are not covered by this remedy in the Materia Medica will, disappear because the etiology, if strong and outspoken, surpasses any other element in the search for the simillimum. *So, don't overemphasize the symptoms if the etiology is clear.*

Sometimes a small change in diet (omitting sugars or dairy products) makes all the difference in the world. As another example for patients who have not been well since an operation, you should consider prescribing Staphysagria. Sometimes the family history may also give a clue to this lack of response. If you find cancer or TB in the family history, sometimes a remarkable improvement is seen in stalled cases with a dose of Carcinosum or Tuberculinum.

119. **Following ghost etiologies:** (another frequent mistake of the beginner); A ghost etiology is one that did not produce any symptoms. For instance, the patient had a heartbreak situation or took a high quantity of Penicillin, but the patient did *not get sick within a year after this event.* Apparently, the Vital Energy of this patient was strong enough to overcome this negative impact. No prescription for this event is necessary: you would chase only ghosts. There was no depression of the Vital Energy. I have said within a year of the event, but usually you can see the symptom production much more quickly after the event; within days to weeks.

For instance, the patient had a flu and was never well since. Or, she had a hysterectomy and has been fatigued ever since. Usually it doesn't take a full year for this clinical picture to appear.

120. **Ignoring the chronology and the layers:** This is so easy to do. Nowadays, psychotherapists are quickly jumping back to the infant stages of the patient. If they suspect child abuse in the patient's history, they jump on it and are surprised that the patient reacts adversely: the shock is too much to be absorbed by the already affected Vital Energy. Often I have seen a patient in my office after such a "healing session" in a state of shock, terrible fatigue and total emotional upset. This is not good therapy, for it has suppressed the Vital Energy. If the homeopathic physician treats a patient, he will carefully take him back from the present time to the time of his birth, constructing a timeline. In this timeline, he notes every event that was intense enough to create physical or emotional symptoms, because that constitutes a layer. And he will start treating the *last* layer first, just like you would peel off the layers of an onion.

For instance, a 25-year-old patient consults with a history of head trauma, causing headaches. Prior to that, there was a breakup, which kept the patient depressed, withdrawn, and unable to cry for one year (age 21). From age 3 to 10, she grew up in a very abusive family in which the father was a dictator. The last layer is the traumatic one and requires Arnica or Nat. Sulph. The next remedy will be for heartbreak, possibly Nat.-m. Only when the symptoms of these remedies have disappeared will we come to the first layer, which is the abuse layer of the childhood, requiring Staphysagria. If you would treat the second layer before the first one, you most likely will have no effect. The remedy is not able to penetrate this first layer. So, go step-by-step; success will be insured. Don't jump over these different layers, because that emotional trauma years ago was very strong. Few adults have only one layer (fewer than 2%). If they do, it shows the strong Vital Energy of the patient. One constitutional remedy will be enough in such a case.

121. **Predetermined hierarchy:** Although I expressed in Paragraph 72 the value of symptoms, common sense should always dictate your prescription. If someone comes to you with a sprained ankle, he will ask for immediate relief. You don't care at that moment if he was abused as a child. Ask the patient, "What is the most important symptom you have today?" As you get to know the patient better, he or she will open up to you and it will be easier to get honest answers regarding their mental state. Few patients will tell you on the first visit that they are jealous, or obsessive compulsive, or that they have a sexual aberration. But as you gain their trust, you will get a more complete picture of the patient. The general rule is to always start with certain symptoms which are *well marked in the patient.*

122. **No underlining of symptoms:** At the time the physician does his intake, he should, underline with one, two or three lines the patient's complaints. Three underlines (or use "3" in parenthesis after the symptom) indicates a strong, outspoken symptom. Two is less intense, and one denotes present but not very outspoken; hence less important. For instance, after a fright a patient with liver symptoms will need a fright-liver remedy. By indicating the intensity of the symptoms in figures 3-2-1, when the physician later reviews the chart, he will have a guideline for his prescription. He will perceive immediately what needs to be cured, what is important to the patient.

123. **Overemphasis of healthy symptoms:** Do not aim a remedy at healthy symptoms. If the patient is romantic, good-natured, responsible, and idealistic, these are healthy symptoms. Separate them from the sick symptoms which constitute the leakages of the patient which need to be remedied first. This makes me think of a case I had in practice. This patient became clairvoyant after a head trauma. In fact, he was so good, he made a living of his clairvoyance. It would be a mistake from my part, to treat the head trauma, since it could take away his psychic abilities, something the patient valued. It is also important to mention that the patient exhibited no negative effects from this trauma.

124. **Prescribing for the name of the disease**: While it is good to have a certain differential in your prescribing after taking a case, we must not forget, as we expressed before, that each remedy can cure any given disease, no matter what it is called. Just prescribing Rhus Tox. for a rheumatic case because it is called a "rheumatic remedy" is the wrong approach and similar to Western prescribing. It could well be that Sulphur would cure that case and not Rhus Tox. ! To say that Sepia is just a "woman's" remedy and therefore never giving it to a man or baby, is another misconception. You are treating a person with rheumatism, not the rheumatism. It bears repeating!

125. **Too frequent repetition:** This is a major stumbling block for the beginner. Again, refer to Paragraphs 50, 53, 54, 57 and 88. Carefully follow their instructions.

126. **Too hasty prescribing:** You can't be too hasty with your prescription, beginner or not. If you go to a lot of trouble with a case (when you know how), it will give you very little trouble afterwards. Conversely, if you have fouled the clear

waters with the wrong prescription, trouble will be endless. If you are not sure, give *Sac. lac.* and study the case.

127. **High potencies in advanced cases:** In advanced cases, malignant or tuberculous, with extensive tissue change or lowered vitality, the worst thing you can do is give your patient the indicated remedy in high potency!! Do just the opposite! Use LM or 6C.

HOMEOPATHIC CASE TAKING

128. To the homeopathic physician, the clinical picture becomes a living portrait of the symptoms of a remedy. Only in this way is the homeopath a good clinician. His approach to disease is primarily symptomatic and only secondarily diagnostic, whereas the allopathic point of view is just the opposite, and symptoms only have meaning insofar as they confirm or support a diagnosis. No account is taken of the vast number of symptoms that may have a modifying influence on the clinical condition per se. Hence, the homeopathic dictum that "*there are no diseases, only sick people.*" For the purpose of prescribing, the *name* of the disease is of little importance.

129. Taking a case is not just noting symptoms as the patient recounts them to you. One of our first concerns is try to find out *where the energy leaks are.* If we are not sealing these leaks, we are losing Vital Energy due to a trauma, a poor diet, a continuous stress factor, bad habits, etc. Why is the patient behaving this way? What motivates him to continue bad habits, even though he is aware of them? Sometimes it is overambition such as the case of the Nux Vomica person who is an executive and has a million things to do, finds no time for relaxation or proper nutrition, neglects every aspect of a

balanced life. Ulcers might be a result of this life-style. Sometimes it is vexation leading to low self-confidence, which is common in the Lycopodium patient, who becomes bloated after eating even small amounts of food, desires sweets and fresh air, is averse to onions and has great performance anxiety.

130. The homeopath takes his case with much greater care than other physicians do. He must observe conditions far more intensely than the allopaths. Many regular physicians scarcely listen to their patients, and, if they report unusual symptoms, brush them aside as if they were purely imaginary. Many believe that the statements of patients are not as important as the evidence obtained with the latest laboratory methods. But in order to make a homeopathic prescription, the most important facts relating to the patient must be discovered, not by scientific examination, but by careful interrogation. Whether a homeopath will succeed or fail in curing his patients, depends largely on the way he takes the case. It is like the difference between a portrait done by Rembrandt and a caricature quickly scribbled by a sidewalk artist.

131. Dr. H.C. Allen, one of our famous homeopathic forefathers, said that a case well-taken is nine-tenths prescribed for. If you have a full and well-taken case, you have little difficulty in finding the proper remedy. Homeopathic prescriptions are built on facts. It is better to have two or three facts that you know are absolutely certain than to have pages of symptoms that are more or less doubtful. You can't afford to have doubtful things enter into a prescription.

132. Homeopathy involves the study of the patient and the remedies and is accomplished by accurate and detailed case-taking. This task is usually exciting and lively. People may

be difficult to understand, contradictory, strange, and hidden, traits we encounter every day in our clinical practice, but there's always a person there to unify the whole picture. It's unified in them even if it doesn't make much sense while that person sitting in front weaves their story, but in the end, it can be an almost perfect match.

133. **Observe and be perceptive** should be our first rule. For the homeopath, the approach to the case is very different from other approaches, such as the allopath's, in that it requires great attention to detail. We are dealing with a whole person, not just the skin or the joints. Consequently, we have to learn how to gain information about the whole person, not just part of the body. A helpful way is to go out to the waiting room to greet the patient. One patient will be calmly waiting for you, reading a book. Another one will be fuming at you because you are ten minutes late. Another one will be happily talking to other people. A child might run around and tear up your waiting room or cling anxiously to his mother's skirt, hiding from any stranger.

You shake the hand of your patient and you note cold and clammy or hot or dry hands. Is this always the case, or is it because the patient is anxious? Is the patient walking briskly or limping? Some patients slouch down into their chairs Or, possibly the the patient does not want to sit down, claiming that he is more comfortable walking around. Or maybe the child climbs on everything it can, touches everything, hums and sings, or goes and hides under the examination table.

Some patients constantly tap their feet, wring their hands and anxiously look around. You should observe whether the patient is well-groomed or untidy, unwashed and smelly. The physician should note the patient's complexion, and whether he has greasy skin, skin rashes or acne, warts, cysts, greasy hair, alopecia, etc. What essential information, what gems to make a prescription, and you haven't even asked a question. Observe the attitude of the patient (calm, quiet, belligerent), note any unusual odors, the patient's reaction to the temperature of the room (wants the windows open, wants the airconditioning turned off, puts on extra clothing, some patients even bring an extra blanket because they feel it is always too cold in the examination room). Observe his mood: Is he worried, anxious, angry, timid, irritable, etc.? The physician's senses have to be educated to be perceptive or he may miss these valuable external signs.

134. The main purpose of the allopathic consultation is to establish a pathological diagnosis, to label the disease in the most up-to-date manner. Western medicine teaches that without this diagnosis, no treatment should be attempted. The investigation of objective pathological symptoms is absolutely essential, according to their beliefs. It is looking for the end-products, the results of the disease. If these results are still not manifested in a precise objective manner, and if the sick person suffers from functional problems only, his case is arbitrarily decided. Either the doctor tells him to come back in six months (hoping he will get sicker and something will manifest itself so he will look like a winner), or he will diagnose it is a nervous, psychological, or imaginary disorder! CFIDS patients, does that ring a bell?

135. But in the homeopathic consultation, we are not satisfied with this investigation *only*. Its object is to establish how a disease was able to establish itself in an individual, to explore all the possible details of the evolution of such a disease in the victim and how precisely *this patient differs from all the others bearing the same diagnosis (individuality)*. Many details, seemingly of secondary or no importance to the allopath, will allow a precise diagnosis of the disease,

especially the diagnosis of *this* patient, and a particular remedy, different from the ten other cases with the "same" disease picture, will be prescribed by the homeopath.

136. The physician must be receptive, like a photographic plate, ready to receive the image of the patient. He must clear his mind of other preoccupations and of previous opinions about the patient. He must be tranquil, cordial, and after the initial greeting and the question "What brings you to see me?", he must be silent. Silence <u>is</u> golden, especially in the beginning of the inquiry.

137. Questions must be asked according to the purest principles of homeopathy:

❑ Avoid direct questions, questions which the patient can answer with a yes or no. Don't ask, "Do you crave sweets?" Instead, ask "What do you crave?" Don't ask, "Are you thirsty?" Instead, ask "What are your drinking habits?" The most reliable information is obtained if questions are posed so that a yes or no answer is impossible. The patient must state the answers in more detail.

❑ Never ask a question which puts an answer, so to speak, into the patient's mouth. You don't ask, "Are you anxious about your new job?" "Are you chilly?" This will bias the patient's answer.

❑ Avoid questions which require the patient to choose between two different alternatives. You shouldn't ask, "Do you prefer sweets or salts?", or "Are your menses clear or dark?"

❑ Distinguish the relative importance of symptoms, place poorly marked symptoms in brackets, and underline (1, 2 or 3) the important ones.

The physician should say as little as possible, try to keep the patient talking and help him stay close to the point. Some patients have to be guided carefully, as the loquacious ones will take you on an elaborated tour of their lives. Others, e.g., Nat.-m. types, will have to be prodded to say anything at all! The process can be like pulling teeth. But never allow yourself to hurry a patient. Establish a fixed habit of examination and stay with it. The last thing you want to do is suggest symptoms to the patient. A suggestible patient trying to impress the physician will respond positively to all your questions regarding symptoms.

138. We have four concerns regarding patient interrogation:

(a) On what basis are the questions to be asked?
(b) What is the best classification to adopt in interrogation?
(c) How should we formulate the questions?
(d) How are we to know if the questions are correctly asked?

(a) Has already been discussed. We have to follow the homeopathic rules and philosophy, considering the patient as a whole and not the sum of his parts; not the pathology, but the living, feeling and thinking patient.

(b) Throughout homeopathic history, beginning with Hahnemann, different classifications have been proposed. Nevertheless, the broad lines converge in the same direction: first, the mental symptoms; then general; then, cravings and aversions; then sexual symptoms, including menstrual cycle; and then sleep and dreams; and finally, the local symptoms related to the organs. Much has been discussed about this in Paragraph 72. Practically, though, in the interrogation it is best to start with the chief complaint (CC), with all its modalities. Then ask other, general symptoms: digestion, thirst, weather-preferences, is the person chilly or hot, perspiration, vaccinations, operations, etc.; then ask about sleep, cravings and aversions, menstrual cycle; and finally the psychological symptoms. By that point, the patient might open up to you and will be more comfortable answering these intimate questions. But the order of questioning does <u>not</u> change the value of the symptoms as we explained in Paragraph 72. Numerous psychological symptoms are clear to the good observer without a word being uttered: timidity, loquacity, easily offended, embarrassed, haughty, immoderately laughing, etc.

(c) After the patient has had time to express his main complaint (CC) without interruption, you may say: "I have listened carefully to you; let's change roles and I would like to ask you more precise questions. I might interrupt you when I have obtained the answer. This just means that a longer explanation would give me neither useful nor new details." This will allow you more control over your time. Otherwise, you might be able to see only one patient a day, which is not very practical. Next, you start formulating various questions to fill in the gaps. You cross-examine the patient to clarify, verify and amend the sensations, locations and modalities described by him.

(d) There are two methods by which to ascertain the effectiveness of the cross-examination.

❑ During the interrogation, the physician must carefully watch his patient and observe the way he answers. Observe the intonation of his voice and expressions, especially his mouth and eyes. Are they looking you straight in the eyes? The eyes are the windows of the soul and will give you a lot of information. Notice how the patient describes his fondness of chocolate and determine whether it is a real craving: the sparkling eyes of the patient and delightful intonation reveal his genuine crush for foods.

❑ During the interrogation, the physician should carefully write down his patient's answers. He should underline the patient's answers. And he should go into more detail if it is an important symptom, just to make sure the patient understood the question correctly. For instance, if the patient tells you that he hates greasy food, you might ask: " Do you prefer fish with sauce or fried in butter?"

It is important for a good physician to be able to make his patient laugh or cry during the initial consultation. Then he knows that he touched the patient, that there has been real contact, and that he has been able to create an atmosphere of confidence and benevolence, which will make his work easier. So often patients told me at the end of the consultation: "Doctor, I already feel so much better, and I haven't even taken the remedy." Could it be that just by being an unbiased but interested observer I had already increased their Vital Energy?

139. To clarify the classification and determine which questions to ask, refer to the following list.

■ *General symptoms:* Statements that begin with "I" or "my"; hourly, periodic, or seasonal aggravations; changes of weather; tendency to catch colds; desire for or aggravation by air; aggravation due to position; riding in cars; prandial aggravations; wounds slow to heal; bloating with localization; bowel habits; hemorrhages; chilly or hot person; reactions to vaccinations; operations; laterality (which side is affected); reactions to fog, sunlight, warmth in general, drafts and wind, being in the mountains or by the ocean; ask about their living conditions and environment; family history (will help to determine miasms).

■ *Mental symptoms* :

❑ Symptoms related to death and suicide.

❑ Ailments due to grief, vexation, indignation, anger, bad news, disappointment in love.

❑ Anger, impatience, irritability.
❑ Sadness, weeping, effect of consolation.
❑ Self-confidence, jealousy, absentmindedness, low self-esteem.

Also ask: "How do people close to you describe you?" and "What complaints do people who know you well have about you?"

■ *Aversions and Cravings:* sweets, pastries, fatty foods, fried foods, salty foods, breads with or without butter, chocolate, coffee, greasy rich foods, alcohol (beer, wine or hard liquor?)

■ *Sleep and dreams:* position of body, causes of sleep interruptions, mental or physical restlessness, time of awakening, reasons for awakening, theme of recurrent dreams.

■ *Menses and sexual sphere:* time of menarche, time between menses, duration, color, clotting, abundant or sparse flow, heavier during day or night, PMS, frequency and regularity, masturbation frequency, sexual habits. The general aggravation of symptoms before, during or after menses is of greater importance than the question of early, late and excessive menses.

■ *Rare, strange and peculiar symptoms:* indicated by the patient with their modalities-- the time it occurred, type of pain, the nature of any discharge, what makes it better or worse.

140. A good homeopath has to include other forms of diagnosis:
❑ *Etiologic diagnosis*: determining the true triggering cause and possible maintaining causes; keep in mind the words *why, when and how.*

❑ *Chronic miasmatic diagnosis*: making a miasmatic diagnosis is setting the patient up for a real cure and eradication of this "taint" so that further generations are free from it.
❑ *Personality diagnosis:* this is the description of peculiar constitution, cravings and aversions, environmental and food sensitivities, etc. It will distinguish the patient from other human beings.
❑ *Therapeutic diagnosis:* depending on the symptoms gathered in the inquiry, taking into account the value of the symptoms.

141. With respect to the *location* of a complaint, it is a good idea to let the patient point to the area of discomfort. You will be surprised to find that the stomach disorder is really a liver problem, or a heart problem is an intestinal disorder. Don't assume that the anatomical knowledge of your patient is the same as that contained in your medical books.

142. When you ask about the *sensation* of a complaint, give the patient the opportunity to describe in his own words, as thoroughly as possible, exactly how it feels. "Like what?" "As if..." Some are imaginative enough to give you an excellent description; others might be helped by some analogies. "Is it like the stinging of a bee?" "Is it burning and itching or burning and stinging"?

143. Taking an *acute case* is different from taking a chronic one. Most of the above rules apply to taking a chronic case. First of all, make sure you have an acute case. You will find that many patients come to you as their last resort, after taking many presription drugs over a long time. Your first prescription should be Nux Vomica or Carbo Veg., antidotes for these modern sins. Most of your acute cases will be taken in a busy, crowded office. It goes like this: "By the way, Doc, my wife just came down with a sore throat. Anything you

can do?" Or: "My child kept us up coughing during the night. Please help us get a good night's sleep." There is often no time for lengthy interrogation, so, you will have to go with what we refer to as a *"three-legged stool"* method. Three sound symptoms are sought and used in the selection. Most important are location, sensation and modality of the chief complaint. Of course, if the patient throws you a keynote symptom of a remedy, you are fortunate indeed. Homeopaths must be instantly ready and willing to take on acute cases and to arrive at the indicated remedy quickly. It helps keep the physician's mind sharp, and will show the power of homeopathy.

144. Also, keep in mind that acute symptomatology will temporarily cause chronic symptoms to abate or disappear. The latter will reappear after the acute illness has run its course. This follows the law that two dissimilar diseases cannot coexist: the stronger one suppresses the weaker one. This has given a false sense of security to CFIDS patients, who claim that their immune system must not be that bad since they never get a cold. But the strong chronic condition (CFIDS) suppresses a minor condition such as a common cold.

145. Why do we homeopaths pay so much attention to emotional symptoms and assign them so much value in choosing a remedy, while Western medicine assigns them little importance, often using them to label the "psychosomatic"?

This is one of the greatest sins of Western medicine and reflects a total lack of knowledge of the natural laws of healing. There is a *centrifugal* flow of disease from within outwards, first affecting the *inner man* (mind, emotion, and intellect), as denoted by a change in his personality. These may be termed the "symptoms of the individual," or the inner dynamic plane of the human economy. The inner man is *always the first to be sick* before the disease filters into the plane of the human economy and into the plane of the physical body. The next group of symptoms to emerge on the surface are disturbances in the functions of the physical body (*altered physiology*). These are chiefly felt subjectively by the patient. This followed by organic and structural changes in tissues and organs, i.e., pathological formation (*altered anatomy*). These are mainly elicited by the physician and detected by our laboratory tests. The last to be affected are the vital organs, such as the brain, heart, kidney, lung, etc.

146. The previous paragraph is extremely important. The "preventive" medicine of allopathic medicine is based almost completely on pathology: the yearly check-up, the Pap smear, the mammogram, the ECG, etc. In other words, what modern day physicians call "preventive" is the last stage of the disease, not the first. This inability to recognize early changes to deal with them has lead to the pandemic of cancer and other immuno-suppressed diseases. Notice this progression of symptoms in a sick child. First, there is a change in disposition (irritability, brooding, either craving consolation or rejecting it, etc.), followed by subjective symptoms: "I have pain in my tummy," "I feel like I want to vomit," etc; then objective symptoms like fever and reddish throat, followed by organ symptoms such as ronchi on the lungs. Western medicine often waits untill the last moment to diagnose and prescribe. Homeopathy is capable of diagnosing and treating in the early stage, often aborting the disease before it progresses. That is real preventive medicine.

147. By far the greatest sin in allopathic medicine is the constant *suppression* that takes place. By suppression I mean that a disease manifestation is disappearing before the disease itself is cured. Alas, this is nothing new, as

Hahnemann so explicitly describes in his Organon, Paragraphs 201 and 202:

"The local affection, however, is never anything else than a part of the general disease, a part transferred to a less dangerous (external) part of the body..."

and

" If the old-school physician (read: modern doctor) *should now destroy the local symptom by the topical application of external remedies* (our modern creams, suppositories, coagulating and lasering), *under the belief that he hereby cures the whole disease, Nature makes up for it by rousing the internal malady and the other symptoms that previously existed in a latent state side by side with the local affection; that is to say, she increases the internal disease."*

Often the first manifestations of an internal disorder develop on the externals, i.e., the skin and the mucous membranes (the internal skin).

148. Medicine is, or should be, the divine art of "healing," and in taking the Hippocratic oath, a doctor swears that he will use his skills, according to his ability and judgment, for the welfare of the sick. For the "sick," mind you, not for the welfare of the pharmaceutical companies or for the stockholders of drug and vaccine manufacturers, who seem to run practically the entire medical profession, except for the brave few who see beyond this and full of divine discontent, dissociate themselves and search for the truth, wherever it may be found.

What a joy it is to find these truths in the old books left by Hahnemann and his disciples, truths which help us heal precious human beings who are burdened not only with original sin, but with the sins of their ancestors. Such chronic diseases are difficult to cure. It is easy enough to suppress, hide or cover the external manifestations of disease by modern methods of treatment. But the original disease remains, and will break out again and again in other areas of the body. And neither the afflicted person nor the treating physicians will see the connecting thread. It is ridiculous to think that by removing eruptions by external applications or operations, one can remove the actual disease that led to those eruptions.

149. Numerous examples of Western suppression of disease can be found. Anything that has been lasered or burned (warts, polyps, etc.) comes back, if you are lucky, since Nature tries again against human "better" judgment, to push the disease out of the body. How many cortisone creams (this poison is available over-the-counter!) have been tried in vain to eradicate poorly understood rashes. How many children got asthma after being treated with cortisone creams for eczema? Western medicine accepts this alternation as a "fait accompli," yet this therapeutic act is actually *causing* it.

Vaginal discharge is another favorite for medical suppression. The suppositories and creams used to treat it are nothing but a therapeutic act against the natural flow of cure. Treatment should be directed at eliminating, and therefore, increasing this flow, since the body tries to get rid of toxins. Even in breast cancer treatment (or other cancers, for that matter), we often see the same thing. Patients who undergo mastectomy with radiation and chemotherapy, often come down with, a couple of years later, a spread of the tumor to the liver or other organs. "We were too late," proponents of this therapy will claim. Has anyone ever stood still and looked at this and reasoned that the suppression of the cancer was so powerful that the only choice was the invasion of other organs?

150. The most constant symptom of many consecutive suppressions is a slowly developing, but steadily progressing, exhaustion of the nervous system, accompanied by low blood pressure, digestive weakness and symptoms of melancholia. The most difficult patients to manage are the new ones, who don't yet understand what they must *not* do: they must not suppress an eruption or discharge which the homeopathic remedy has been trying to elicit. Warn your patients that they should do nothing and explain Hering's Law to them.

151. We have other kinds of suppressions which are not due to medication, such as suppression of strong emotions, more or less conscious suppressions which can lead to illness. There is also suppression following acute grief, mortification, or indignation. There is a kind of natural suppression, such as the cessation of after getting wet, cold feet, or perspiration inhibited by chilling. Another form of suppression follows the "Law of Dissimilars:" *a severe acute disease can suppress the chronic disease until the acute disease is cured.* Suppression is not the privilege of Western medicine alone. A homeopath often finds that certain symptoms are relieved by his remedy, and yet the patient feels worse or develops more deep-seated problems. In this case, the prescribing has been superficial and suppressive or at best, palliative, if it was an incurable case.

152. A homeopathic case taking is not complete without a thorough *physical examination.* This examination often reveals facts the patient willingly or unwillingly forgets to mention. I remember a case referred by another homeopath in which the patient complained of a stinging pain around the anus, "as if a splinter had penetrated my skin." Numerous remedies had had no effect. When I examined the area, there

was a splinter embedded in the skin. Removal of it cleared all the symptoms. How embarrassing if you miss something like that. Often the patient does not mention rashes until you observe them (or warts, cysts, lipomas, etc.).

153. *Common sense* should overshadow the other senses in case taking. It helps us to determine whether the symptoms are to be our guide or whether we should treat them as pathognomonic symptoms. Hahnemann further urges: "Fidelity in noting down the image of the disease. The physician will need this image for further reference and study and to determine the progress of recovery." The patient relates the story of his illness in his own words without interruption, and what he fails to mention, family members communicate as best they can. Here we must sit in judgment to determine what will be helpful to us. The patient is so used to relating common symptoms such as, "I am so fatigued," "I have muscle and joint pains," which do not mean much until we get the modalities as to location, time, aggravation, sensation, amelioration, etc. It is rare that we spontaneously get a guiding symptom. Keep in mind that some people do not observe their symptoms. This is dependent not upon their education, as some of the most well-educated people are the worst at relating symptoms. It depends more on their innate ability to see, and feel, and then relate to others.

154. Another class of patients are those who exaggerate all their symptoms, the true "hypochondriacs." The latter is not a demeaning word, as it so often is in allopathic medicine. The typical Arsenicum, Nitric acid and Psorinum patient is very concerned with his health, feels that he will die no matter what you do and is therefore, the most difficult to treat. Even when there is improvement, he will tell you there is none.

This exaggeration alone is a guiding symptom and will lead you to the remedy.

155. A good inquiry requires the physician to be four people at once: It requires the sound wisdom of a judge on the bench and the sagacity of a philosopher. At the same time, it should be conducted with the tenderness of a mother and the exactness of a mathematician. This careful and painstaking process will reduce the work of your prescription to a minimum. At the end of your case taking, write down an *assessment*, a short paragraph containing your thoughts about the case, how you see the different layers, and what remedy you will try first, with at least one or two back-up remedies in mind. If, over the next couple of visits, the first remedy does not work out, you will already have two others ready. Plan which remedies you will give for the different layers you observed. Write down the present miasm(s).

156. Summary: In order to take a good case we must be familiar with the *"Five Knows of Homeopathy."*

- ❑ KNOW PATHOLOGY *etiology *diagnosis *prognosis
- ❑ KNOW REMEDIES *dosage *provings on the healthy
- ❑ KNOW HOW TO ADAPT REMEDY *Like Cures Like *totality of symptoms*single remedy *minimum dose
- ❑ KNOW OBSTACLES *constitutional *diet *living conditions *occupational hazards *surgical blocks *psychological barriers
- ❑ KNOW HOW TO DETECT EARLY DEVIATIONS and treat them early

MANAGEMENT OF THE PATIENT

157. There is something that every homeopath learns very quickly in the beginning of his practice: the importance of the **second** prescription. Most of us think the initial prescription requires all our skill and intelligence, yet a good clinical result depends mainly on the second prescription. A quick, irrational follow-up of the case can easily spoil all the fruits of your hard labor in the first consultation. You may only call a prescription the second one if it follows a first one that has *acted.* Only when we are able to do a first prescription that produces perceptible changes (physical and/or emotional) in the patient can the subsequent prescription be called a second. Wrong prescriptions are not termed prescriptions at all. So, the accurate interpretation of the changes occurring after the remedy has been given is, in some respects, more important than the selection of the drug and the repetition of the dose. Kent goes even further when he says, "*The whole future of the patient may depend upon the conclusions that the physician arrives at after the remedy has been administered.*"

158. **What are possible scenarios following the first prescription?** Understanding each of these will keep you on the right track. No matter how much the patient wants to change a remedy, or thinks it is not working when old symptoms recur, you, the physician who is well-versed in the field and has the integrity to continue to study, must be the guide of the ship. How often have I seen on my telephone slips, "I am no better" yet when I talked to the patient, I found that there had been significant improvement. The patient, being used to the Western Houdini disappearing act of drugs, called suppression, misunderstands the

reappearance of old symptoms, increased discharges or rashes, or initial similar aggravation (aggravation of existing symptoms).

159. *Immediate improvement without any aggravation* is the first and best observation. The patient feels a sense of well-being, his sleep pattern improves, sensitivities decrease, clarity of mind returns, symptoms disappear and calmness prevails. It is positive proof that the potency was not too high, but just high enough to cope with the ailment from which the patient is suffering. If there is an improvement of 50% the first week, the golden rule is *slow down*! If you don't, you inevitably will steer towards an aggravation. Do fewer succussions (in the case of LM) or start taking the C potencies less frequently (once a day, or every other day). The patient needs to take the remedy as infrequently as possible while still holding a gradual level of improvement. This immediate improvement without aggravation also means that the disease was not deeply rooted (no organic changes).

160. *No reaction:* there is neither aggravation nor improvement, even after two to three weeks. Why?

❑ Possible wrong remedy, but often we will see new symptoms appearing.

❑ Before you change the remedy, especially when you think the prescription was well-indicated, change the potency! Go from 6C to 30C, 200C, or 1M.

❑ There might be a miasmatic block that prevents the indicated remedy from working: Recognize the miasm and prescribe the indicated anti-miasmatic remedy.

❑ Something in the life-style of the patient either cancels the remedy or is a maintaining inciting cause of the disease (poor environment, continued abuse of tea or coffee, continued alcohol use, bad eating habits, etc.). Review the history with the patient again. Often you will hear, "I was really doing better until I started drinking every day." This roadblock should be removed before making any change in the homeopathic remedy.

❑ Patient is sluggish in reacting (see Paragraph 161).

161. *Initial improvement, then return of the symptoms as they were before the medicine was given.* Possible reasons:

❑ The first to be entertained is that it was the right remedy but apparently the stimulus from the remedy is not strong enough to sustain improvement: first try increasing the potency.

❑ Possible presence of a miasm; needs to be removed first.

❑ The prescribed remedy was similar (the simile) but not the simillimum. A new prescription is needed because the first prescription was not the real totality.

❑ Review the life-style of the patient (see Paragraph 160).

❑ There might be a structural change in the organs; they may be damaged beyond repair and, we can do only palliation. In these instances, an increase of potency would only harm. One always has to be on guard for hidden and unrecognized pathology.

This reaction is often seen in violent, rapidly progressing acute diseases, where the power of the medicine is used up quickly by the intensity of the disease process and frequent repetition is necessary to produce a curative reaction. It is also observed in sluggish, phlegmatic individuals (Calc. Carb. types) who are slow to respond to the action of the best selected remedy. In such cases, use high potencies (1M or 10M).

❑ We must not forget to wait awhile in chronic cases, as the Vital Force has cycles; true curative action must not be interrupted until it is certain that the reactive force is exhausted; **watch and wait!**

162. *Quick similar aggravation followed by improvement and increase in the patient's strength:* this indicates an excellent prognosis; the remedy was well chosen and the improvement will be long lasting. In this case, there is no tendency to organic change and the prognosis is good (curable case). An aggravation of this sort is seen mostly in patients with strong vitality and good reactive power, but it is also frequently seen when the potency used was higher than necessary. A lower dilution would have avoided the aggravation. Some homeopaths claim that this scenario has to be achieved or no improvement can be expected. However, it is within the experience of every careful observer to meet with cases where relief and nothing but relief, has promptly succeeded the administration of the well-selected homeopathic remedy, relief so rapid that it seemed almost like magic. A gentle reaction always leads to a more permanent cure. Aggravations are rarely more than a few hours in acute diseases, several days for chronic diseases (with low potencies and in non-sensitive patients).

163. *A long continued aggravation but final and slowly progressing improvement:* this reaction occurs when the medicine was administered in a potency too high for the reactive power of the patient, whose vitality, however, was able to assert itself and, in time, genuine curative action begins. It is usually an indication that the case was on the borderline of incurability and often where extensive pathology is present. Do not repeat too soon, but wait until the patient has sufficient strength to react to another dose.

164. *Prolonged aggravation and slow decline*: if the remedy was well-chosen, the case was simply incurable because of the marked irreversible organic changes. You can only hope for palliation by zig-zag prescribing. In other words, you are changing the remedy as the need arises in the acute situation,

the acute symptomatology being your guideline. You need to select low potency remedies (not beyond 30C) of a palliative nature in doubtful and incurable diseases. It happens rarely, but in this case, it could also mean that the potency was too high for the feeble reactive powers of the patient.

165. *Immediate improvement, short-lasting:* (same as reasons given in Paragraph 161); if you see a sharp aggravation after an initial improvement in an acute case, it indicates that the inflammatory process is too violent, and the second prescription should be a frequent repetition of the same medicine in higher potencies: from 30C to 200C to 1M; this is the case in desperate, acute conditions.

166. *Aggravating reactions to every remedy:* this illustrates the case of the "hypersensitives." They are the most difficult to treat but make the best provers of the remedy. As mentioned before, high potencies should be avoided at all costs in these cases. Use LM or low C potencies (6C). Other possibilities: the patient has serious unmet emotional needs, and other family members should be interviewed to clarify the case. Use placebo and concentrate on the psychological symptoms.

167. *Symptom improvement, but no relief and no special increase in the strength or mental condition of the patient:* the case is incurable; the physician can only palliate. This is always the case in scarring and partial destruction of the organs. The remedies act favorably, but there is only so much they can do. The remedies may keep the patient comfortable, and by careful repetitions at frequent intervals the patient may be kept comfortable for a considerable period of time, although you shouldn't expect a cure because of the extensive pathology. Other possible reasons for this situation: the potency was not correct to complete the action

started, or else toxic environmental factors are interfering with the action of the remedy. Check the home environment.

168. *Rapid amelioration of the symptoms, followed in a longer or shorter period by a long aggravation:* this is an unfavorable reaction. Either we did not choose the simillimum (but the simile) and, therefore, the remedy acted only as a palliative, or the disease is incurable. Don't change your remedy too hastily. Some remedies have a deferred aggravation. Phosphorus is one of them (up to twelve days). Also, if the severity of the aggravation and the nature of the symptoms belong to the so-called external parts of the body--skin, mucosae, joints--while the mental and organ symptoms improve, by no means should a change of remedy be considered. In chronic cases, aggravations may come and go like waves, even until the fourth month.

169. *Longtime improvement, then sudden aggravation:* in this scenario the patient starts proving the remedy and shows accessory symptoms or symptoms of the remedy. It means that the patient is almost cured. You should stop the remedy and wait. The aggravation will disappear and the patient will stay in an improved state for a long time. Only when symptoms start reappearing should a single dose of the previously indicated remedy be given, and this should be followed by immediate improvement. Accessory symptoms can also appear when the remedy was unnecessarily repeated.

170. *Symptoms follow Hering's Laws*: puzzling to the patient, but what a joy to the physician, who knows a real cure is establishing. Here we should just watch and wait, for the same remedy will continue the improvement. Prognosis is good if the case is not interfered with. However, if you see superficial symptoms disappear, only to be replaced by organ

symptoms, stop the remedy immediately! It is the wrong remedy. The disease is going in exactly the opposite direction of Hering's Laws. For instance, there is an improvement of joint symptoms, but the asthma is aggravated. As Kent expressed: *"To prescribe for rheumatic conditions without due regard for the other symptoms of the case is dangerous. To fit a remedy to one part or organ may jeopardize the future health or even the life of the patient."* The oldest ailments, among which are the constant local ailments, are the last to give way. When old symptoms come back, the psychological are the most important and the best guide for the selection of the remedy.

171. *New symptoms appear:* the symptoms are neither old symptoms reappearing (often called new symptoms by the patient) nor the symptoms of the remedy prescribed (similar aggravation). This is a *dissimilar* homeopathic aggravation, indicating a wrong remedy. There might be an exception to this rule. There is a class of new symptoms which indicate that the remedy is acting curatively. It may be the moaning of a comatose patient who is returning to consciousness or the marked tingling in a paralyzed part when the motor and sensory nerves are again beginning to function. A new symptom such as leukorrhea never experienced may be a favorable sign under the action of the well-chosen remedy. The unexpected appearance of an eruption on the skin is an indication that it had been suppressed and the patient had forgotten to mention it.

172. When remedies are used with intelligence and precaution, it will be very rare that the physician has to *antidote.* The only time this would be indicated is when you did not recognize a hypersensitive patient and you started with a high potency.

173. If, during the course of the treatment of a chronic illness, an acute disease appears, stop the selected chronic remedy and prescribe the indicated acute remedy. When the acute situation subsides, continue the chronic remedy as before.

174. Mental improvement is an outstanding indication of favorable remedy reaction. Sleepiness after a remedy is also a positive sign, indicating that the remedy is acting deeply.

175. If a patient does not react to the well-prescribed remedy, use a nosode. Through its deep penetration into the life spirit, a nosode is endowed with the power to stir the defective vitality to a state of reaction, or may bring latent symptoms into open expression so that the proper remedy can be applied and convalescence and a complete cure achieved.

176. It is quite possible to treat an acute phase of a chronic case (which is a mistake) and feel that progress has been made only to find that suppressed symptoms begin to appear. Detoxification can be done too rapidly. The patient feels infinitely worse than before the treatment was started and you'd better have a good explanation or the patient will lose heart. The toxins can be released in such large quantities that the liver, kidneys and skin are unable to compensate for the increased load put upon them. This is analogous to hasty homeopathy and needs to be avoided.

177. There are also some objective criteria of improvement after the intake of a remedy. The first one is the *body temperature*. The drop of temperature in an acute case is an indication that we can stop the remedy, as the remedy has taken hold of the case. Further continuation would have only a counter effect to the first few doses and possibly harm the patient. Take the temperature under the arm, as the oral is

far more changeable and less practical. Normal axillary temperature is 97.5F. Any persistent temperature rise in a chronic case, no matter how slight, always leads, in time, to degenerative diseases.

A second objective criterion is the *heartbeat*. Heartbeats remain increased as long as the temperature is above 97.5F. The third one is the *blood pressure* measurements. If a patient had a blood pressure of 90/60mm and after the remedy it rises to 110/80mm, then the remedy was the simillimum. The hypertension of adults, if on the simillimum, is always normalized, regardless of age.

178. Whenever a frequent change of potency is necessary, the medicine is likely the simile rather than the simillimum.

179. Although not generally recognized in homeopathic circles, many types of therapy are accompanied to a greater or lesser degree by aggravations. Among these are acupuncture, osteopathic manipulations, colonic irrigations, massage, fasts or other diets, and psychotherapy.

180. When my patient is better, Nature has taken charge. I let her alone. She is a better doctor than I am. More cases are bungled by too frequent repetition than by anything else. As Kent says, "*Sac. lac. is the second-best remedy.*" It is wise to give the patient plentiful placebo or Sac. lac. along, similar in appearance to the actual remedy. This is especially important for patients who are used to taking a lot of medicine.

PALLIATION AND INCURABLE DISEASES

"A physician can only save a patient not destined to die."
(Japanese proverb)

181. The real use of palliation, which is temporary relief of symptoms, is in the case of so-called *incurable* cases. The root of the tree is too sick to be cured and therefore an attempt is made to cut only the branches. Alas, palliation is misused greatly in modern medicine, for several reasons, partially, because doctors confuse palliation with cure. They use palliation over and over again in curable diseases until the case finally becomes incurable because of suppression of symptoms and consequent involvement of internal organs. Another reason for overuse of palliation is the patient. Sometimes they don't understand the difference between a cure and palliation and demand immediate relief, by any means. They don't think about possible side-effects or creation of worse diseases. The examples are numerous in modern times. In "Suppression of Symptoms," we discussed the devastating therapeutic modalities in rashes, discharges, warts, cysts, etc. So a strong factor limiting curability is the *tolerance of the patient and the patient's family.* The symptoms which may arise during the curative process may be too difficult to tolerate because they are too intense, misunderstood or socially unacceptable. Homeopathic treatment may take longer than the rapid elimination of symptoms by allopathic drugs. Social and peer pressure often lead to a return to ineffective allopathic treatment, but that has the glow of "speedy symptomatic relief" written all over it.

182. Homeopathic physicians can make the same mistake. Many homeopaths practice homeopathy in a Western way: they cover a few symptoms in their prescribing, but neglect the totality, one of the cornerstones of homeopathic prescribing. The physician goes from one remedy to another, always temporarily ameliorating some symptoms, but never curing the patient. This happens when the physician is too busy to do a good inquiry, or when he succumbs to the wishes of his patient to prescribe something "for the rash on my fingers." The remedy may offer temporary relief and improve the rash, but then it reappears after three months. This is because all the pertinent data were not taken, and another remedy, the simillimum would have removed all the symptoms of the patient, not just the rash. That's why the combination remedies are so popular. This shotgun approach, severely condemned by Hahnemann, results in palliation at best. But unfortunately these so-called "homeopaths" do injustice to the patient and harm the profession of homeopathy. Correct prescribing is an obvious requirement for homeopathic effectiveness.

183. Where is palliation indicated?
❑ In cases with irreversible and structural damage such as advanced cancer cases, nephritis, nephrotic syndrome, advanced M.S., optic nerve atrophy, etc. One word of caution here. So many cases which have been declared incurable by orthodox medicine have become curable after judicious employment of the LM potencies of the indicated remedy. The reason for this is that the Western diagnosis, based on pathology, physiology and knowledge of internal medicine, cannot determine the exact state of the Vital Energy. A good example of palliation in homeopathy is the administration of Arsenicum 200C to a dying patient. It relieves the immense anxiety and restlessness and makes the patient's final hours more comfortable.

❑ In cases where organs are removed, for obvious reasons: after removal of a kidney, stomach, part of bowel, spleen, etc. Many of these cases, though, could have been spared the operation in the first place if treated according to the root of the problem, not just the branches.
❑ In cases where the Vital Force of the patient is too weak and he cannot withstand the stimulus of the prescribed remedy.

184 The previous paragraph should help convince the homeopath not to pursue obviously incurable cases, except for the purpose of palliation. Otherwise, we homeopathic physicians would harm the patient by offering false hope, leading to contempt for the physician and homeopathy alike. But there are certain methods, helpful in less obvious cases, to ascertain the incurability of a case. Some, we already discussed in the "Management of the Patient." What are these signs?

❑ After the correctly indicated remedy, the homeopathic aggravation continues for a long time and the general condition of the patients continues to deteriorate.
❑ After application of the indicated remedy, there is quick, short living amelioration, followed by aggravation (cancer is a classical case).
❑ If the amelioration after the homeopathic aggravation does not persist, and no obstacle to the cure can be established.
❑ If some of the symptoms improve but the patient does not regain a sense of well-being.
❑ If after a well-selected remedy, the symptoms follow a path contrary to "Hering's Laws."

185. Palliation by means of homeopathy is of the greatest value, but cannot always be carried out, due to the conditions of the patient. Surgery, aside from traumatic or structural surgery,

relates mainly to the removal of pathological end-products, which frequently threaten the usefulness, comfort and the very life of the patient. Under such circumstances, nothing else can take the place of surgery.

186. If you treat successfully an acute condition with a 30C potency, then most often you can prevent the recurrence by giving the same remedy in 6C or LM potency. How long a remedy will work, depends on the thickness of the layer to be treated. It has nothing to do with the remedy itself.

SECTION TWO

"When one ceases to think and read, one has reached the deadline and is well on the road to mental decay."

CLINICAL CONDITIONS

☞ **<u>NOTE:</u>** In this section of the book, different clinical conditions are discussed with their homeopathic remedies. A good homeopath will keep in mind that for any given condition, <u>any</u> given remedy can be indicated as long as it is prescribed according to the homeopathic laws and principles outlined in Section One. However to make its application easier for the beginning and busy practitioner, this section discusses clinical conditions with their main indicated remedies. Using the third part of the book, the "Materia Medica of Musculoskeletal Diseases", the practitioner will be able to make a differential diagnosis between these remedies while acquiring a working knowledge of the main remedies used in his practice. Hopefully, it will stimulate him to study further and discover the power and expansive knowledge that homeopathy has to offer.

FRACTURES

It speaks by itself that common sense has to prevail when a fracture is suspected. All the first aid has to be applied, X-rays are taken to assess the damage, bone setting has to be done properly and proper shock treatment is instituted.

But there is much to do homeopathically. If the fracture is extensive enough or the traumatized individual is sensitive, the first homeopathic remedy coming to mind is ***rescue remedy*** in tincture form to alleviate shock. Everyone should have this remedy in the practice, at home and in the car. 10 drops in water should be given immediately repeated q. 15' if necessary. Next, a closed, "simple" fracture will require **first** ***Arnica*** to help the bruising, the pain and the shock. After a few days, ***Ledum*** will complete the work of Arnica. Only after the bone is set, ***Symphytum*** will be given. The latter is really the orthopedic specific of the herb remedies. When there are many fractures at the same time, after rescue remedy and Arnica, ***Silica*** will be indicated to renew the "edifice sand", to increase and rebalance the grit and stamina of the person.

An open or *"compound"* fracture has to be attended surgically, of course, but after the surgery, ***Calendula*** 200C, one dose for three days will help heal the wound. When there is injury to nerves, ***Hypericum*** will be used. Afterwards, the same remedies as for the closed fracture will apply.

Fractures in children are usually less complicated than in adults and will require the same remedies. There is one unfortunate incident in which fractures are common or where the physician will discover fractures in different stages of healing: the *"battered child."* In this case, after the fractures have been attended to, ***Staphysagria*** 6C or LM1 will be needed to restore the indignation the child had to endure.

In case of fractured ribs, where the slightest movement of the respiration will hurt, ***Bryonia*** will bring relief. In case healing of fractures is slow in spite of Symphytum--as sometimes happens with aged patients--, ***Calc-p.*** will speed up the process. It favors the formation and calcification of callus.

Another type of fracture, often seen in unconditioned athletes, is the *stress* or fatigue fracture. It usually occurs after long hikes, after running while not in condition, overexertion and repeated strain. ***Arnica*** will be very helpful. If this is seen in children who grow too fast and who exhibit growing pains, ***Calc. Phos.*** will be their healing and constitutional remedy.

BRUISES AND BLACK EYES

In the treatment of bruises caused by trauma causing muscular ecchymoses of the soft parts, ***Arnica*** always comes first to mind. There is simply nothing better to speed up the absorption of blood (that's why it is used as a first remedy in stroke) and to alleviate the pain. Use Arnica internally and externally for fast results. If the pain seems to be located deep in the bone, use ***Ruta.*** If there are no rapid results with Arnica, Ruta or Rhus Tox, try ***Conium.*** If the wound was not well attended to and suppuration set in, a few doses of ***Hepar Sulph.*** will stimulate the suppuration.

☞ Note: spontaneous bruising without trauma may indicate ***Sulphuric Acid***

"Black" eyes caused by blows from a fist or sport accidents like a tennis ball in the eye, require ***Symphytum*** as the #1 remedy. ***Ledum*** is the #2 remedy. Ledum in general follows Arnica very well when the ecchymoses have turned violet-black. ***Staphysagria*** if the black eye comes from anger or rage during a fight.

Note: ***Coccus cacti*** to remove an insect, dust particle or any foreign object from the eye.

HEAD TRAUMA

"Never well since" (nws) a head trauma" is a strong etiology. In practice, often I have seen debilitating disease resulting from a blow to the head, fracture to the head in an accident and concussion in general. CFIDS, memory disturbances, character changes, recurrent headaches, and vertigo attacks are some of the few consequences I have noticed. But no matter what the symptoms are (they could be

constipation since the head trauma), if it is "nws head trauma", the following remedies have top priority.

The first one to consider will be ***Arnica*** again. Often it will revive the patient (in case the patient is stuporous, give the remedy in water and put a few drops on the lips, q. 10'). A second remedy, often indicated, especially when the spine is involved, is ***Nat.Sulph.*** Nat. Sulph. is also indicated if we see change in mental functioning after a head trauma. Also, use Nat. Sulph. when Arnica only palliates. ***Hypericum*** might come in handily if the radiating, nerve pain persists.

BURSITIS

Definition: inflammation of the bursa, which is present wherever a muscle or tendon moves over a bony prominence.

Etiology: infection, trauma.

Symptomatology: swelling, redness, local tenderness and sharp pain on any movement when infection takes place.

Homeopathic treatment: ***Apis*** is the main remedy; ***Ruta, Bellis-Perennis, Rhus Tox., Silica and Bryonia*** are the other remedies. Silica will be last to speed the healing process.

NECK AND CERVICAL SPINE

CERVICAL DISC SYNDROME

Definition: irritation of one of the eight pair of nerve roots arising from the cervical spinal cord. Most occur at the C5-C6 level which corresponds with the irritation of the sixth nerve root.

Etiology:
- ❑ acute trauma
- ❑ cervical arthritis with spur formation

Symptomatology: when nerve irritation is involved, tingling and numbness is often noted in the forearm and shoulder on the side of the pinched nerve; morning stiffness is possible, sometimes going to severe torticollis where the slightest movement will be worse and the neck is frozen with pain inasmuch that the patient does not want to be touched. Trigger point tenderness is often present together with a weakness of the muscle group innervated by the irritated nerve root.

Prognosis: if properly treated very few will require surgery; the latter should not be imposed on the patient unless no improvement is seen after several weeks and MRI shows clear pinching of the nerve. The homeopathic remedies speed up the recovery dramatically.

Homeopathic therapy: ***Arnica, Rhus Tox., Hypericum, Nat.Sulph. and Bryonia*** are the main remedies.

The first remedy is often Bryonia, because the patient is in so much pain, that he does not want to be touched (massage or manipulation). The next choice will depend on the modality that is predominant: Rhus tox. for the extreme stiffness, Hypericum for the tingling and numbness, Nat.

Sulph. if the cervical spine is much involved and Arnica only palliated. Keep ***Ruta*** in mind if the patient comes to you after a bad manipulation or over-manipulation.

WHIPLASH

Definition: hyperextension of the soft tissues in the neck, classically caused by a rear-end car accident. The brutal force of the trauma is absorbed by the ligaments and muscles which can be severely stretched.

Etiology: rear-end collision.

Symptomatology: amazingly enough, often immediately after the trauma few symptoms can be noted. The patient will say, "there is nothing wrong with me." Usually, hours later or the next day, stiffness will set in leading to a certain degree of torticollis with limitation in movement. With time, an X-ray will show the reversal of the normal cervical lordosis (a straightening of the normal curve).

Prognosis: early treatment is the key, even if the symptomatology is poor in the beginning; it is sufficient to have the classical trauma to start treatment immediately. To the amazement of the patient, often none of the above symptoms appear if the adequate remedy is prescribed.

Homeopathic therapy: one dose of ***Arnica*** 200c will help with the shock of the patient who claims, "nothing is wrong" with him. The next remedy often, because of extreme pain (depending on the intensity of the trauma), will be ***Bryonia.*** As the pain decreases, ***Rhus Tox*** . ideally is indicated to help restore the soft tissue injury and mobility. ***Hypericum*** in case of nerve involvement with tingling.

TORTICOLLIS

Definition: there is a painful rotation of the neck with tilting of the head to the opposite direction.

Etiology: it can be congenital, traumatic, or secondary to an inflammation, spinal cord tumor or cervical spine abnormalities (osteophytes). We will discuss mainly the traumatic and inflammatory torticollis.

Symptomatology: painful spasm of the neck with an opposite tilting of the head. Stiffness can be outspoken, limiting any movement of the neck severely. This can lead to frontal headaches and exhaustion.

Prognosis: the traumatic and inflammatory forms can disappear inasmuch as a few hours to a few days. Spinal abnormalities need to be ruled out by X-ray and MRI if there is no fast improvement with the well-prescribed homeopathic remedy.

Homeopathic therapy: ***Lachnanthes (#1) and Causticum*** are the main remedies. Other remedies are: ***RhusTox., Cicuta and Cuprum.*** These remedies can be used for both forms of torticollis, but there is one outspoken remedy for the inflammatory torticollis. The latter is usually caused by exposure to extreme and sudden cold, such as chill dry wind or the child (or adult) getting sweaty while playing outside without toweling himself immediately. The result is often a stiff neck or an intense fever the next day. There is only one remedy which brings immediate relief: Aconite. Rhus Tox. usually finishes these cases.

THORACIC OUTLET SYNDROME

Definition: it is a name given to four different syndromes. Cervical rib, scalenus anterior, costoclavicular and hyperabduction syndrome all have in common neurovascular compression at the base of the neck. The most common is the cervical rib syndrome. The clinical findings among these syndromes are almost identical.

Etiology: a cervical rib arising from the seventh vertebra pressing on the neurovascular structures.

Symptomatology: pain and numbness, especially in the hand and the inner aspect of the forearm; also tingling along the ulnar nerve, weakness causing the patient to drop objects, and coldness are common symptoms.

Prognosis: operation is rarely indicated unless conservative treatment (ultrasound and exercises) fails. The pain and inflammation is usually quickly relieved with homeopathic remedies.

Homeopathic treatment: ***Hypericum, Rhus Tox., Causticum, Graphites*** are common remedies. Graphites covers tingling, numbness and pain very well. Hypericum for outspoken nerve pressure symptoms will often be the first remedy, while Rhus Tox. will show a definite aggravation in damp weather.

THE SHOULDER

SUPRASPINATUS TENDINITIS

Definition: inflammation of the rotator cuff muscle (most commonly the supraspinatus) tendons.

Etiology: repeated trauma causing inflammation and thickening and aging. Typical lesion for a pitcher in baseball.

Symptomatology: sharp, electrical pain with a locking sensation as "if the muscles and tendons are too short," especially in abduction. Worse with pressure, stiffness can be present because of spasms of the muscles. Lameness.

Prognosis: operation is only necessary when there is a complete rupture of the rotator cuff muscles, resulting in total loss of motor function.

Homeopathic treatment: ***Causticum, Arnica, Ruta, Rhus Tox., and Sanguinaria.***

Rhus Tox. and Sanguinaria will be major remedies here which is not surprising looking at their modalities: tearing, rheumatic pain on motion, lifting the arm, turning in bed, stiffness, in damp weather, etc. "Feeling of tendons too short" responds well to Causticum.

TENOSYNOVITIS OF BICEPS TENDON

Definition: inflammation of the tendon of the long head of the biceps.

Etiology: overstraining of the muscle like in throwing, playing tennis while serving and overuse of the limb like in lifting heavy objects or reaching up too high for something.

Symptomatology: external rotation with abduction leads to a very sharp pain, restricting the motions of the shoulder. Sensitive to pressure (cannot lay on the affected side), better in rest.

Prognosis: very favorable with conservative therapy; cortisone shots should be avoided.

Homeotherapeutic treatment: ***Rhus Tox (#1) and Ruta*** are the main remedies. In the beginning, if pain from the slightest movement, ***Bryonia*** and ***Arnica*** will help. Ruta has a particular affinity for the periosteum. Arnica is useful in the primary stage of the injury. *What Arnica is to contusions, Rhus Tox. is to strains.* In almost every case where there is over-stretching of a part, especially ligaments and tendons, Rhus Tox. will help.

FROZEN SHOULDER

Definition: as its name says, complete restriction of shoulder movement which is "frozen."

Etiology: while Western medicine blames tendinitis, I have seen it often after sleeping in awkward position, overuse and over-extension of limbs (I had a conductor of an orchestra with bilateral capsulitis), in housewives before the Christmas period who get all "tensed up" because of the approaching holidays with increased responsibilities and family reunions. This anxiety usually caused an epidemic of frozen shoulders in my practice. Another exiting factor is internal adhesions post-surgery.

Symptomatology: the onset can be gradual but I have seen it often occur overnight. The shoulder is immobilized and very little movement is achieved if any, under sharp, excruciating pain. Especially, trying to elevate the arm or coaming the hair is impossible, while lying on the affected side is avoided because of pain.

Prognosis: while recovery is slow in Western medicine, I have treated and cured frozen shoulders in a matter of days or weeks with acupuncture and homeopathic remedies.

Homeopathic therapy: ***Thiosin (#1), Rhus Tox., Ruta, Ferrum, Bryonia*** and ***Sanguinaria*** are the main remedies. Thiosin or mustard seed oil will be used in 3x or 6x potency. It is an excellent scar remedy and used to prevent internal adhesions after surgeries. Rheumatic pain with lameness. Bryonia gives the extreme feeling of dryness, "as if there is no synovial fluid in the joint." Sanguinaria for right shoulder affections.

DISLOCATIONS

Definition: most commonly *anterior* dislocation; the humerus is lifted from its glenoid cavity into an anterior position.

Etiology: mostly directly from a trauma (fall) on the abducted arm.

Symptomatology: easy to diagnose because of the prominent acromion and the limitation of movement because of the severe, bruised pain. Numbness can be present.

Prognosis: usually easily to reduce with gentle straight traction with counter traction applied to the axilla without general anesthesia.

Homeopathic therapy: after the reduction, give first a dose of ***Arnica 200C.*** It will help with the bruised pain and the shock. The next days, ***Ruta or Rhus Tox***. will finish the work of Arnica.

Patients under the age of 30 have a great recurrence of dislocations. ***Calc-p, Silica, Kali-c or Calc.carb.*** can help when prescribed constitutionally.

☞ **NOTE:** Shoulder pain does not result always from direct pathology of the shoulder. Often, internal pathology, especially referred shoulder pain from liver disease, subphrenic abscess, gallbladder and pancreas disease has to be considered. Diaphragmatic irritation can also come from internal abdominal bleeding after trauma. In homeopathy, we have several remedies with a specific keynote, referring to the shoulder-blade. The best well-known is the pain felt at the *lower corner of the right shoulder-blade.* It relates to the remedy, ***Chelidonium,*** a liver remedy. These patients have a strong desire for warm drinks and food, a strong dislike for cheese and an inability to digest fats. The presence of this dull or lancinating pain at the shoulder-blade location is a super keynote, enough to prescribe the remedy.

A keynote for ***Phosphorus*** is the presence of a burning spot *between* the scapulae. ***Lycopodium*** has the same burning feeling between the shoulder-blades. Note that these three remedies are all liver remedies. So one should be highly suspective of liver pathology with "shoulder pain, non-related to shoulder pathology."

ELBOW

TENNIS ELBOW

Definition: inflammation of the tendons mainly of the extensor muscles at the lateral epicondyle (exterior tennis elbow) or the flexor muscles at the medial epicondyle (interior tennis elbow, less common).

Etiology: it is mainly an "overuse" of the limbs; its name is derived from a frequent lesion in tennis, when beginners mishit the ball, or when switching to a different racquet and strings with different tension, causing additional strain on the tendons where they attach to the epicondyle. Of course, it is not only restricted to tennis buffs. Overuse of the arm while painting a ceiling, carrying heavy objects, or repetitive twisting movements can easily cause this epicondylitis.

Symptomatology: sharp electrical pain, very sensitive to pressure. The pain is present when shaking hands with someone, or when lifting a cup of coffee, or simply when

\writing. The pain radiates in the forearm, mostly following the Large Intestine meridian in Acupuncture (Heart meridian in the interior tennis elbow). Local tenderness on the epicondyle.

Homeopathic therapy: ***Ruta*** is the #1 remedy because of its affinity for the periosteum and ligaments, with pain consequential to repeated strain. If Ruta does not help, ***Bellis Perennis*** is a deeper acting remedy. Other remedies are ***Anacardium, Arnica, Agaricus, Aurum Met., Rhus Tox.(#2!), Hypericum and Bryonia.***

☞Note: remedies acting according to depth: Arnica----Ruta----Bellis Perennis---Millefolium----Hammamelis

OSTEOCHONDRITIS DISSECANS

Definition: is an avascular necrosis of the subchondral bone, also often seen at the knee joint, leading sometimes to separation of part of the bone, which can then float around in the joint.

Etiology: most likely traumatic.

Symptomatology: dull, aching pain with a certain degree of stiffness, worse in the morning and in first movement, improving with slow movement but getting worse again if overexerted. There is local tenderness and sometimes joint swelling because of effusion.

Prognosis: early cases will respond quickly to homeopathic remedies. Surgery is only required if recurrent locking occurs, necessitating the removal of the floating particle.

Homeopathic remedy: the majority of the cases will respond well to ***Rhus Tox.*** Once there is redness, tenderness and effusion, ***Apis*** will help. If a trauma was the onset of the problem, then first ***Arnica*** should be considered. It will stop the case from progressing.

OLECRANON BURSITIS

Definition: inflammation in the olecranon bursa.

Etiology: direct acute trauma.

Symptomatology: in the acute phase there can be tenderness, formation of blood in the bursa sac and limitation of the movement. In case of infection, all the classical signs will be present: tenderness, redness, swelling, and pain with the slightest movement.

Prognosis: proper treatment should prevent chronicity.

Homeopathic treatment: the first few days, **Arnica** will be given, followed by ***Ruta*** to finish the case. In case of infection, first ***Bryonia*** followed quickly by ***Hepar Sulph.*** to help with suppuration. ***Apis*** in the beginning stage of inflammation.

FOREARM AND WRIST

CARPAL TUNNEL SYNDROME

Definition: a compression of the median nerve, often bilateral (50%).

Etiology: often the cause is not clear although it has been found in higher incidences with hypothyroidism and arthritis. Repetitive trauma as in certain extreme wrist movements could cause inflammation and pressure on the median nerve. Holistic doctors have been able to give relief with Vit B6, which does not mean automatically there was a deficiency of this vitamin in the first place.

Symptomatology: pain at night, with numbness and tingling over the median nerve course up till the middle finger; there can be weakness, lameness, numbness, improved by letting the hand hang down or shaking it. My patients often use to tell me that they must have "poor circulation" since their symptoms subsided by moving the hand.

Prognosis: it is my conviction that early homeopathic treatment could avoid a lot of operations. Only motor weakness with beginning atrophy should warrant surgical cutting of the transversal carpal ligament.

Homeopathic treatment: ***Guaiacum, Mag-p, Ruta, Caust., Hyper., Rhus Tox. and Calc-p*** are the main remedies. Once the patient comes to you with the carpal tunnel syndrome established, Causticum will be your first choice. The #2 will be Mag.-p. In the early stages, when the symptoms just come up (like early weakness while writing), then Ruta will be your choice. When the wrist is very stiff, swollen and "cracking" is heard, Rhus Tox. is indicated.

Guaiacum for right-sided carpal tunnel in a person craving apples.

GANGLION CYST

Definition: is a cyst containing mucinous material, very common in the dorsum of the hand but may occur anywhere else in the body.

Etiology: unknown. Trauma?

Symptomatology: sometimes none at all, except visible when flexing wrist especially. Deep localized cysts might pressure tendons and cause dull persisting pain, worse in movement.

Prognosis: most people tolerate these cysts without any intervention. Some want something done for esthetic reasons.

Homeopathic treatment: a cyst is part of the sycotic miasm. Therefore ***Thuja*** is the #1 remedy if other signs of sycosis are present. If inflammation is present, ***Bryonia*** will bring relief.

DUPUYTREN'S CONTRACTURE

Definition: progressive contracture of the palmar fascia, leading to a flexion deformity of the distal portion of fingers, often bilateral.

Etiology: unknown, more in males.

Symptomatology: there is no pain; the finger is gradually pulled into flexion; often the ring finger is first affected while other fingers follow.

Prognosis: in order to avoid surgery (fasciectomy), early treatment is necessary.

Homeopathic treatment: ***Causticum, Cuprum, Nux.Vomica, Secale, Plumbum and Mag-p.*** Causticum (#1) and Mag-p will be the front runners. The same remedies will help in the "*Trigger Finger Syndrome*" in which a swelling of the flexor tendon hinders the passage through the sheath. This results in a painful snapping, worse after rest, improved with movement. Again, Causticum overall is the first remedy to try, especially if other symptoms of this remedy are found in the suffering patient.

ULNAR NERVE PARALYSIS

Definition: paralysis of the ulnar nerve at its most superficial location behind the elbow.
Etiology: chronic trauma.
Symptomatology: paresthesias and numbness in forearm and hand (also dorsum); there is no limitation in movement and no night pain.
Homeopathic treatment: ***Hypericum, Ruta and Arnica*** . Arnica and Ruta in the early stages right after trauma, Hypericum when the paresthesias have become apparent.
In later stages ***Aconite, Calc. Carb., Graphites and Rhus Tox.*** can be of help.

Some cases might require surgical transferal of the nerve, especially the ones linked to recurrent subluxation.

SPRAINED FINGER

Definition: inflammation and swelling of the distal joints.
Etiology: trauma, especially sport trauma.

Symptomatology: painful swelling of the metacarpal phalangial joints, restricting movement, with possibility of blood collection in the joint.

Homeopathic treatment: ***Arnica and Rhus Tox.*** Start with one dose of Arnica 200C, the next day continue with Rhus Tox. 30C till improvement. Resolves the situation in 2 days most of the time. An excellent method is to take one dose of 30C, 200C and 1M with four hours interval. Then wait.

BITES

Definition: we refer here to human and animal bites.

Symptomatology: the biggest danger is of course the inoculation of virulent oral bacteria into the wound.

Homeopathic treatment: our first concern will be avoidance of infection. Therefore ***Calendula 200C*** orally will be given, as well as applied locally in a watery solution on some gauze. Then ***Hypericum*** will be our first choice, followed by ***Ledum.*** These last two are the first choices for cat bites. For dog bites, Hypericum is #1 while ***Belladonna*** (with infection signs) and ***Lyssin*** (potentized saliva of a dog with rabies) are indicated, especially if one suspects and wants to avoid rabies. Hypericum is also the #1 for bites of spiders, scorpions, rats, and insects.

☞ NOTE: **Ledum** is #1 for flea bites, followed by ***Staphysagria*** and ***Pulex irritans*** which is nothing else than the potentized flea. This is very effective for dogs and their flea bites.

PARONICHIA or PANARITIUM

Definition: a Staphylococcus infection of the distal phalanx of the finger along the edge of the nail.

Etiology: caused by a cut or a bite or biting off the nail.

Symptomatology: all the signs of local infection (tenderness, redness, swelling); pulsating, sharp pain "as if a blood stream jets through the finger."

Homeopathic treatment: ***Anthrax, Hepar Sulph., Silica, and Apis*** are the main remedies.

Anthrax will be number one, especially when there is a burning feeling. If this is not available, Apis will be given when there is stinging pain with much swelling and redness (first phase of panaritium). Once there is yellow pus, first Hepar Sulph. will be given since it brings the pus out. After this, Silica will speed the healing process. All this can be accomplished in 1 to 2 days so drainage and antibiotics can be avoided in the majority of cases.

RAYNAUD'S DISEASE and PHENOMENON

Definition: attacks of vasospasms, usually bilateral in women mainly; the Raynaud's phenomenon occurs in the course of other disease such as scleroderma.

Etiology: unknown.

Symptomatology: the spasms in the fingers or toes cause first pallor, followed by cyanosis and hyperemia. There is a painful tingling and a cold formication feeling. Triggered by cold or emotional stress, especially worry about the past and anger.

Prognosis: I have seen very few good results with Western medicine and small areas of gangrene can occur if the condition becomes chronic.

Homeopathic treatment: ***Agaricus(#1), Sepia, Hypericum, Lachesis*** and ***Secale.***

Agaricus will always be tried first since it has the typical cold formication symptom with constriction and crawling feeling. Secale is more for formications on the tip of the fingers and threatening dry gangrene. ***Lachesis*** when there is gangrene with blue/purple skin and oozing of pus and blood. For scleroderma ***Graphites and Calc. Carb.*** can be indicated.

PHANTOM PAINS

Definition: very painful condition occurring sometimes after amputation of a limb.

Etiology: irritation of the regrowing nerve ends at the stump

Symptomatology: severe burning pains, hypersensitivity, painful prickling feeling.

Prognosis: Western medicine has very little to bring relief except the heavy duty painkillers with their addictive effects. I treated a case on Demerol, with acupuncture only with excellent success. However, acupuncture combined with homeopathy is capable of bringing relief to the majority of the cases, avoiding the toxic drugging effects of modern medicine.

Homeopathic treatment: ***Coffea and Allium Cepa*** are the major remedies. ***Hypericum and Calendula*** are the other remedies. ***Staphysagria*** and ***Aconite*** are last resort remedies when the above have failed.

Coffea covers the severe burning pains and hypersensitivity while Allium Cepa is indicated in the painful prickling sensation.

TRUNK AND SPINE

LUMBAR DISC SYNDROMES

Definition: extrusion of the disc into the neural canal, also called sciatica.

Etiology: repetitive trauma causes degeneration of the nucleus pulposus; Arthrosis deformans and degeneration of the disc can lead to similar symptoms. Rarely occurs in children and up to the twentieth year. Oftener in females than males. The gouty and rheumatic diatheses exert an undoubted influence in the predisposition to sciatic neuralgia. A strongly marked nervous temperament, exposure to cold and dampness and direct injuries to the nerve by blows and falls are more common exciting causes.

Symptomatology: most disc lesions occur between L4-L5 (follows the external gallbladder meridian in acupuncture) and L5-S1 (follows the bladder meridian along the back of the leg). While acute events of sudden pain may occur, usually the disc patient has manifested at intervals low back pains, aggravated by bending forwards or backwards, after sitting down for a long time, causing a certain degree of stiffness, worse with sneezing and walking, or improving with walking, and heaviness and weakness in lower back. As the situation becomes worse, radiation down the leg occurs with decreased sensation in the leg and foot. Limitation of movement is obvious in different degrees. Soreness along the course of the nerve is observed, usually sensitive to pressure. Coldness, or an abnormal heat of the affected limb is often present.

Prognosis: MRI should rule out other causes like spinal cord tumor. Operation is performed too often. In my view it is mostly indicated in the rare *cauda equina syndrome* where there is a massive disc protrusion, resulting in bladder and bowel function disturbances. The circumstances of the patient's life may make a cure improbable, such as exposure to the hostile influences of cold, damp, and privation, or to great mental distress, or habitual maintenance of the sitting posture in business for many hours together; in short whenever the exciting cause continues to exert its influence.

Homeopathic treatment: ***Aesculus, Agaricus, Bryonia, Colocynthis, Dioscorea, Gnaphalium, Hypericum, Kali Iodatum, Mag. phos., Rhus Tox., and Phytolacca*** are major remedies. Following the modalities in the Materia Medica of these remedies results in tremendous, miraculous and fast results. Colocynthis, Gnaphalium, Hypericum and Bryonia especially for the acute cases. ***Sulphur*** , ***Rhus Tox.,*** and ***Arsenicum Album*** for subacute, chronic and more advanced cases. Rhus tox. especially caused by exposure to dampness, or straining in lifting.

I remember a patient who had gone to all kinds of doctors for the last 6 months with no relief. Desperate, he considered an operation but heard from a friend about some cures I effected in other people. He was a typical Hypericum case. While he was undergoing acupuncture I give him a Hypericum 30C. Great was his surprise that the pain was abated completely by the time he left the office. I only needed to see him once more after this. He walked again for miles and did not suffer from backpain till now, 3 years later.

LUMBAGO OR LUMBAR STRAIN

Definition: pain in lower back because of muscular or ligamentous injury.

Etiology: trauma, emotions (especially fear and anger), obesity, lack of exercise, cold-damp weather exposure, suppressed sweating after exercise, bad working habits, lifting weights, working in yard in stooped position for a long time, and hereditary factors such as spine stenosis, spina bifida or spondylolisthesis.

Symptomatology: stiffness, dull pain, worse with bending forwards or backwards, worse with sitting, better with slow movement; fatigue, lameness and tenderness.

Homeopathic treatment: ***Ammon.Mur., Arnica, Colocynthis, Dulcamara, Gnaphalium, Guaiacum, Kali Bich., Kali Carb., Radium Brom., Rhododendron, and Rhus Tox.*** Some keynotes will bring you quickly to the matching remedy. Arnica when overlifting or overuse of limbs; the cramping pains of Colocynthis; the pain in small spots for Kali Bich.; the backache preceding the menstrual cycle with Kali. Carb.; the aggravation of backache before a storm with Rhododendron and the outspoken stiffness with sensitivity to dampness of Rhus Tox. Dulcamara is a back-up for Rhus Tox. Careful examination of the Materia Medica will make the differential diagnosis.

Calc. Carb. (for the obese person) ***and Calc. Phos.*** (for the slender person) can be constitutional remedies for people with a "weak" back and can prevent the recurrence of lumbago.

SKOLIOSIS

Definition: lateral curvature of the spine with a rotational curvature.

Etiology: non-structural (flexible and correctable with side-bending) skoliosis is a compensation to a disc problem or a leg length discrepancy. Structural (non-flexible and not correctable with bending) skoliosis is "idiopathic," in other words from unknown causes and constitutes the majority of skoliosis.

Symptomatology: usually asymptomatic in young people where it will discovered through a school examination. It is frequently seen in the fast-growing adolescent between 11-14 year old (Calc. Phos. type). An X-ray will confirm the extent of the skoliosis.

Prognosis: some will improve spontaneously but it will be difficult to predict acurately.

Homeopathic treatment: ***Calc.-p*** given to children with skoliosis in their growth spurt will be very helpful against the progression of the skoliosis and the growing pains in the long bones. Other remedies are ***Calc. Carb., Calc-f, Phosphorus, Silica and Sulphur.*** Most of these remedies are constitutional and this will be helpful in determining your choice.

If there is pain in the curvature, ***Sil. and Aesculus*** will be our first choices. The same remedies will be used for kyphosis (normal for thoracic and sacral spine) and Scheuermann's Disease (fixed kyphosis around puberty).

BECHTEREW or ANKYLOSING SPONDYLITIS

Definition: also called Marie-Strumpell disease; consists of a chronic inflammation of sacroiliac and spinal joints.

Etiology: more in men, frequently familial although it is seen in women with colitis ulcerosa.

Symptomatology: insidious onset with low back pain and pain in the buttocks; there is extreme stiffness which limits the motion of the spine ("bamboo-spine"); also sacroilical tenderness is noted. The HLA-B27, an antigen marker, is useful to confirm the diagnosis and screen people with a family history.

Prognosis: Western medicine is usually aimed at exercises and anti-inflammatory agents. However, homeopathic remedies will provide better relief without the side-effects and procure in general a normal life-style.

Homeopathic treatment: ***Rhus Tox., Causticum, Kalmia, and Aesculus*** are the main remedies. ***Calc. Carb.*** is the chronic of Rhus Tox. and will be given in a constitutional dose (1M) once the stiffness is under control. Aesculus and Kalmia are the main remedies. Other possibilities are ***Conium, Kali Carb. and Agaricus.***

OSTEOPOROSIS

Definition: common disorder in which the total skeletal mass is decreased.

Etiology: often seen post-menopausal and in elderly patients; often a lack of activity and faulty diets (sugar, fats, fried foods, lack of fiber, alcohol, and an <u>excess</u> of protein [cause #1, not deficiency of protein as Western medicine claims]) lead to osteoporosis. A new study, published in the *New England Journal of Medicine (2-'94)*, showed that cigarette smoking significantly increases a woman's risk of osteoporosis.

Symptomatology: insidious; sometimes a fracture is the first symptom and most of the time it is discovered incidentally on X-rays. Sometimes even so simple a motion as walking or sitting can collapse vertebrae and fracture wrists and hips.

Homeopathic treatment: is safe and cheap and can be instituted before the menopause or immediately after. ***Calc.-p 6x*** , (especially in tall, thin people) will avoid intake of estrogen/progesterone. It will be the #1 for osteogenesis imperfecta. ***Calc. Carb.*** will be indicated in more obese people. ***Calc-f., Sil. and Symph.*** are to be used when failure with above remedies.

BONE CANCER

Definition: we refer here to metastatic bone cancer, coming from the prostate, breast, kidney and lung.

Symptomatology: pain at night not relieved by rest and not responding to the right homeopathic remedy must make you think of it. Advanced cases show complete paralysis with bladder and bowel disturbances.

Homeopathic treatment: ***Phosphorus, Symphytum and Conium*** are the main remedies. Others are ***Cadmium Met., Aur.Met. and Calc-f.***

Conium is especially indicated if the mets come from the prostate, cervix and breast. In case the patient will receive radiation or chemotherapy, its side effects are greatly relieved by ***Cadmium Sulph. 30C***.

HIP AND PELVIS

OSTEITIS PUBIS

Definition: inflammation of the pubic symphisis.
Etiology: trauma, after childbirth or urinary infections.
Symptomatology: local tenderness, aggravated by coughing and bending as well as active adduction of the hip.
Homeopathic treatment: ***Arnica, Bryonia and Ruta.*** Arnica 200C immediately after the trauma while Ruta will cure when Arnica only palliates. Bryonia when the inflammation is established and the slightest movement hurts.

TAILBONE PAIN or COCCYODYNIA

Etiology: trauma (fall on coccyx, during pregnancy), chronic strain and osteoarthritis later on; or neuralgic, which may be of rheumatic or gouty origin. A fall, either coming down in a sitting posture on the ground, particularly on the ice or hard pavement, or on the sharp edge or border of a prominent body, is the most frequent mode of injury. The chronic consequences of a fall are either a malposition of the coccyx sideways (rarely observed), backward, or forward. The latter is the most common.
Symptomatology: sharp, electrical pains, sometimes radiating in the buttocks, aggravated by sitting on a hard seat, local tenderness.
Homeopathic treatment: ***Hypericum(#1), Arnica, Bellis Perennis, Ruta, Rhus Tox., Bryonia, Kali Bich., Causticum, Carbo Animalis, Tellurium and Silica.***

Hypericum, Silica, Bellis-P, Ruta and Carbo Anim. are the main remedies after a fall in that order. With Caust. there is drawing pain, aggravated during menses and evening. Rhus Tox. with outspoken stiffness, stinging like a needle and radiating to the thighs; Kali Bich. in evening and radiating to urethra before urination and while walking.

COXARTHRITIS

Definition: degenerative arthritis confined to the hip.

Etiology: trauma, obesity, and avascular necrosis of the femoral head.

Symptomatology: dull pain, referring to the knee, better after continued movement and heat, worse after rest and in initial movement, upon rising, stiffness, especially in morning; in advanced cases, all walking becomes painful (pinching, pressing, shooting, tearing). Limited movements and sometimes flexion contracture.

Homeopathic treatment: ***Aesculus (#1), Tellurium, Cimicifuga(#2), Kali-c, Rhus Tox. (#2), Colchicine, Medorrhinum, Ledum.***

Aesculus is a major hip and sacro-ilical remedy, very helpful in the weakness and pain on getting up from a chair. As more stiffness develops and rheumatic pain becomes more outspoken, Rhus Tox. is more helpful. Kali-c has also the outspoken weakness with improvement in movement. Colchicine is the gouty arthritis, < on movement (<> of Rhus Tox.) and the least touch, with cracking joint. Cimicufuga is for the hormonal arthritis in menopause.

THIGH and KNEE

MENISCUS TEARS

Definition: a tear in the "C" shaped cartilage, acting as a cushion.

Etiology: typical soccer injury or on twisting movements of the knee with the foot in weight-bearing position.

Symptomatology: well-localized, sharp pain, more common at the location of the medial meniscus; swelling the next day from effusion; after the acute symptoms subside, intermittent dull or drawing pain, radiating to the hollow of the knee; lameness with periods of locking can occur; pain is worse while squatting and walking upstairs. Local sensitivity can persist.

Homeopathic treatment: ***Arnica, Bryonia, Apis, Rhus Tox., Ruta, Calc. Carb., Ruta.***

Calc. Carb. when ascending stairs and squatting; Rhus Tox. worse in rest and upon initial movement and rising from a seat with stiffness and tearing pain; Arnica after the initial trauma followed by Bryonia when the slightest movement is painful; Apis for the swelling and effusion if Arnica and Ruta do not clear it up.

INFLAMMATION

Etiology: trauma.

Homeopathic treatment: ***Apis, Ruta, Rhus Tox., Bryonia***

Apis and Bryonia in the immediate, acute phase while Ruta and Rhus Tox. will finish the case.

LIGAMENT LESIONS

Etiology: forceful trauma against the knee while the extremity bears weight.

Symptoms: swelling localized, bruising, sensitivity, tearing pain, abnormal movements noted when compared with the other knee. If ill-treated, chronic instability of the knee occurs.

Homeopathic treatment: ***Rhus Tox. (#1), Arnica, and Ruta.*** Rhus Tox. will be in all cases the #1, given in three consecutive doses of 30C, 200C, and 1M with four hours interval. Arnica and Ruta can be given in a 200C immediate after the trauma. To strengthen the ligaments afterwards, ***Natrum Carb.*** and ***Strontium Carb.*** are the leaders, while ***Calc. Carb.***, being the chronic of Rhus Tox., will also prevent recurrence, especially in the Calc. Carb. constitution.

RECURRENT SUBLUXATION OF THE PATELLA

Definition: common in athletes, the patella dislocates laterally

Etiology: sport trauma.

Symptomatology: swelling, local tenderness, and a sensation of the knee giving out.

Homeopathic treatment: ***Arnica, Ruta, Apis, Bryonia and Rhus Tox*** for the acute phase. ***Calc. Carb., Phosphorus and Nat. Carb.*** for the prevention of recurrence, according to the constitution.

LEG, ANKLE and FOOT

ANKLE SPRAINS

Definition: stretching or tearing of lateral ligament mainly.

Etiology: trauma, especially sports (like soccer, tennis, football), resulting from an inversion or plantar flexion.

Symptoms: starts usually with mild, dull pain; as times goes by, swelling and pain become more outspoken with functional limitations; of course more severe strains cause immediately the above symptoms.

Homeopathic treatment: ***Arnica, Bellis-perennis, Bryonia, Rhus Tox. (#1) and Ruta (#2)*** for the acute phase. ***Nat.-c and Calc. carb.*** for prevention of recurrence. Old strains which give sequelae such as intermittent pains, swellings and easy relapses: ***Strontium carbonicum***

TARSAL TUNNEL SYNDROME

Definition: pressure on the posterior tibial nerve.

Etiology: injuries, secondary consequences to fractures and deformities of heel and foot.

Symptomatology: burning pain, numbness and tingling in sole of the foot, radiating into the calf. Worse with exercise.

Homeopathic treatment: ***Secale, Caust., Rhus Tox., Sulphur and Silica.***

Secale and Causticum will be first choices.

ACHILLES TENDINITIS

Etiology: overuse of calf muscles in athletes.
Symptomatology: sharp pain, local tenderness, swelling and crepitations.
Homeopathic treatment: ***Rhus Tox. (#1), Ruta (#2), Arnica, Rhododendron, Bryonia, Kali-Bich. and Causticum.***

MORTON'S NEUROMA

Definition: fibrosis of the plantar nerve.
Etiology: trauma.
Symptomatology: severe burning pain in the region of the third web space radiating to the third and fourth toes; numbness and exquisite tenderness between 3rd and 4th metatarsal heads.
Homeopathic treatment: ***Nat.-c, Apis, Aur.-met., Staph.***

CORNS and CALLUSES

Etiology: as a result of abnormal pressure against the skin of the foot, due to improper shoe wear; perspiration causes maceration of the skin.
Symptomatology: hard corns are mostly on the dorsal aspect of the proximal interphalangial joint of the fifth toe; sharp, boring, burning pain can develop.
Homeopathic treatment:

❑ **Calluses:** ***Antamonium crudum(#1), Graphites (#2), Calc. carb. and Silicea.***

❑ **Corns:** ***Ant.-c, Caust., Calc. carb., Rhus-tox., Sepia and Sulphur.***

WARTS

For the homeopath, they are an expression of the miasm, **sycosis**. They respond well to homeopathic treatment and <u>don't need local treatment,</u> unless for psychological reason, when the patient does not understand that the appearance of a wart is an expression of a deeper terrain factor that needs to be treated. In this case, local ***Thuja*** cream can be applied.

Homeopathic remedies: ***Thuja, Caust., Nit. Acid, Dulcamara, Ant. Crudum.***

Caust.: especially for plantar and subungual warts.
Ant. Crud.: horny and hard warts.
Nit. Acid: cracked, easily bleeding warts with nettling pain.
Dulc.: flat warts on back of hands and back.
Thuj.: #1 remedy except for plantar warts, also for moles and papillomata and polyps.

DISORDERS OF TOENAIL

INGROWN NAILS: caused by incorrect nail trimming, tight shoes or bony deformities. ***Graphites and Silica*** are the main remedies. Also ***Caust., Nit-Ac. and Thuja.***

HANGNAILS: ***Sulphur (#1), Rhus-t., Sil., and Thuja.***

INJURIES: for crushed nails, either from hammering on your finger or getting caught between the door, or someone steps on your toe, there is nothing better but ***Hypericum*** to bring quick relief from the burning, stinging nerve pain. Other remedies are ***Arnica and Ledum.***

SPECIAL PROBLEMS

GUNSHOT WOUNDS

Homeopathic remedies: ***Hypericum, Calend., Arnica, Ledum and Gunpowder.***

Hypericum was used in W.W. II and prevented a lot of shock situations. A dose of Calend. to prevent infection.

BONE SPURS

Homeopathic remedies: ***Calc. Flor and Hekla Lava*** are the main remedies. Other ones are ***Aur.-Met., Phos. and Silica.***

Hekla Lava was discovered when goats, eating the lava from a vulcano crater, started to grow exostoses, especially on the jaw. Take a 6C potency, when the exostoses are not painful, a 30C/200C when painful.

OSGOOD-SCHLATTER DISEASE

Definition: involves the tuberositas tibiae of adolescents.

Etiology: most likely traumatic .

Symptomatology: local tenderness and pain, < with walking, exercise and squatting.

Homeopathic treatment: ***Calc-Phos and Silica;*** these remedies are both constitutional remedies and often the constitution will make the choice between the two.

PUNCTURE WOUNDS

Etiology: stabbing, splinters.

Homeopathic treatment: in every case first ***Calendula*** to avoid infection. For intense pain, shock and healing ***Ledum and Hypericum.*** Hypericum especially when the part is lacerated or crushed. Remember that Hypericum is a fine preventive of tetanus. Ledum is the remedy for penetrating wounds par excellence, and for splinters producing pus. Remember that the traumatized part is cold to the touch or maybe the patient feels it cold even while warm to the touch! For pain or headache after a lumbar puncture, use ***Hypericum.*** Stings from insects: wasps ***Apis and Ledum;*** bee stings ***Apis, Ledum and Urt. Ur.;*** jelly-fish ***Apis.*** When hypersensitivity to the pain, patient cannot bear to be touched, ***Hepar Sulph.*** The main remedy for splinters is ***Silicea.*** Give in 200C potency and 1M the same day. Then wait. ***Apis*** is equally good for penetrating wounds where the patient cannot stand that his cloths or sheets touch the lesion. ***Plantago*** is remarkable to relieve the pain very fast in a wound caused by stepping on a rusty nail.

☞ Note: of course, "Tolle Causum" comes first: try to remove the foreign body.

GOUT

Definition: inherited metabolic disease with deposition of urate crystals in cartilage, joints, subcutaneous tissue and bone.

Etiology: exact nature of the disease is unknown; inherited increase of uric acid, mainly men (95%); secondary to leukemia, diet factors (wine, anchovies, sardines, liver, kidney, hering), toxic drugs or decreased renal clearance of uric acid; history of associated complication of obesity and diabetes.

Symptomatology: sudden onset of the acute attack, usually in a single joint (big toe or knee mostly), swelling, redness, heat, starting at night; local tenderness; pruritus after the attack with asymptomatic periods of months or years after initial attack.

Homeopathic therapy: ***Urtica Urens #1, Benzoicum Acid, Colchicum, Ledum, Sulphur, Nux Vomica, Calc. Carb., Aurum-met.,Sabina.***

For the acute phases, Urt. Ur. is first followed by Benz. Ac. and Colch. Urt. Ur. was Dr. Burnett's favorite remedy which he prescribed in tincture form (10 drops BID). It cures more cases of gout than any other remedy by removing uric acid. He kept it a secret as long as he lived and became world-known as the doctor who could cure more gout than anyone. After his death, his daughter shared the secret with humanity.

Note that Western medicine has "borrowed" Colchicine to treat acute attacks. Ledum is excellent for gout of big toe if Urt.Ur. does not work and the patient puts his foot in ice-cold water to alleviate the pain. Aurum-met for chronic gout. Sabina for plethoric women with gouty diathesis and depression.

ARTHRITIS of BIG JOINTS

Definition: we mention here mainly the inflammatory form of arthritis.

Etiology: unknown; the osteoarthritis is related to trauma, heredity and aging.

Symptomatology: stiffness of the joints, with swelling, redness, pain at night and in morning, worse with cold, improved by continued motion, massage and heat; the hallmark of R.A. is a symmetric polyarthritis of the joints; osteoarthritis in contrast, primarily affects those joints that either transmit the body's weight along their axes or absorb repetitive stress and motion.

Homeopathic treatment:

It is a fact that any remedy in the materia medica may be indicated in arthritis. Careful case taking and willingness to thoroughly study the case are necessary.

- ❏ for R.A.: ***Rhus Tox (#1), Calc. carb., Cimic., Dulcamara, Apis, Bryonia, Salicylic Acid, Rhododendron, Ledum, Kalmia, Graphites***
- ❏ for osteoarthritis: ***Actea Spic., Kali-c, Caust. and Guaiacum.***

Kalmia is descending arthritis with wandering pain; Ledum ascending arthritis and traumatic arthritis; Dulcamara is a back-up of Rhus Tox. since it can feel the weather changes (especially damp weather) too; Salicylic Acid is homeopathic aspirin, especially useful for Meniere's Disease; Apis and Bryonia for any swelling with redness and pain in an acute attack; arthritic conditions developing around the menopause call for Graphites.

ARTHRITIS OF SMALL JOINTS

Homeopathic Therapy: ***Actaea Spicata*** and ***Caulophyllum,*** are the main remedies. The first remedy specifically for men, the second for women.

FROSTBITE

Etiology: exposure for a certain duration to cold combined with dampness and a chilling wind factor; can occur quickly at higher altitudes.

Symptomatology: especially nose, hand and feet will be affected; swelling, later redness and sharp twitching pains with possible vesicle formation. Severe forms go to necrosis and gangrene.

Homeopathic treatment: warming up of the extremity should be avoided!! The law, "Like Cures Like" is applicable: use snow first to rub gently on the affected limb. Don't put the patient near a stove, it is sufficient to put him in a room, away from wind and cold. ***Agaricus #1*** remedy; others are ***Silica and Zinc.***

☞ NOTE: Every climber should have Agaricus in his first-aid kit and take a dose preventively. Besides Agaricus, a second valuable remedy for climbers would be either ***Carbo Vegetalis*** or ***Coca***. Both are wonderful remedies for altitude sickness.

HERPES ZOSTER or ZONA

Definition: activation of chicken pox virus residing in root ganglia.

Etiology: any decrease in the strength of the immune system can lead to the reactivation of this virus (emotions, fatigue, other diseases, etc.).

Symptomatology: a period of stinging, burning pain precedes for some days the vesicular eruption; postzonal neuralgias are often persisting in older debilitated patients.

Homeopathic treatment: ***Rhus Tox. (#1), Ranunculus Bulb., Arsenicum Album, Sulphur*** are the main ones. Other ones are ***Mezereum, Variolinum and Apis.***

Mezereum: vesicles with thick yellowish liquid, thick hard crusts with underneath yellow pus. Variolinum will show pustules comparing to the small pox vaccination. Rhus Tox. is by far the #1 remedy, for the zona and the postzonal neuralgias. The modalities of the pain sensation will give the clue to the simillimum.

BELL'S PALSY

Definition: paralysis of VIIth cranial nerve.

Etiology: often seen after exposure to dry cold air (riding in the wind), or after getting wet or trauma.

Symptomatology: paralysis of the muscles of one side of the face with disappearing of naso-labial groove, asymmetry of the face on showing teeth and Bell's Sign in eye on trying to close it.

Homeopathic treatment: ***Causticum #1, Gelsemium, Acon., Nux Vom., Rhus Tox.***

Causticum is mostly indicated in this disorder. Gels. effective in drooping eyelid, Acon. after exposure to dry wind, Nux Vom. when there are a lot of spasms.

REMEDIES INDICATED IN INJURIES FROM THE ANATOMICAL STANDPOINT

Head: Arnica, Cicuta, Hypericum and Natrum Sulph.
Eyes: Symphytum, Ledum, Arnica.
Spine: Hypericum, Arnica, Agaricus, Ruta and Aesculus for S.I joints.
Wrists and ankles: Ruta,(#1), Rhus Tox.
Fingers: Hypericum.
Knee: Ruta.
Ankle: Rhus Tox., Ruta, and Ledum; Kali Carb. and Strontium Carb (for chronic cases).

TYPES OF WOUNDS OR INJURIES

Punctured: Ledum, Hypericum, Nitric Acid.
Lacerated: Calendula, Hypericum.
Contusions and hematomes: Arnica, Rhus Tox, Ruta, Hammamelis, Conium, Symphytum.
Gunshot: Hypericum, Gun powder, Calendula, Arnica.
Incisions (surgical) and stabs: Staphysagria.
Burns: Urtica Urens (1st degree), Causticum (2nd degree) and Cantharis (3rd degree).
Sepsis: Calendula, Pyrogenium and Echinacea.
Infected wounds: Calendula internally and externally.

RECAPITULATION

Arnica: shock, fractures, contusio, stroke, bruises, dislocations, overuse of limbs or voice, and soft tissue trauma
Hypericum: lacerations, and any injury involving nerve endings
Ruta: trauma of periosteum, involvement of ligaments and tendons, and overuse of limbs and eyes
Symphytum: stimulates knitting of the bones
Ledum: puncture wounds, bites, stings, pains improving with cold
Bellis Perennis: deeper acting Arnica, affinity for pelvic area
Rhus Tox.: affinity for ligaments, joints improving with movement; and great stiffness
Actea Racemosa (Cimicifuga): arthritis of the big joints, while **Caulophyllum and Actea Spicata** have an affinity for the small joints.

SPORT TRAUMAS

An excellent way of prescribing for acute sport traumas is one dose of each of the 30C, 200C and 1M with 4 hours interval.

Skiing:

❑ Spraining of ankle will require Arnica, Rhus Tox. or Ruta in acute phase, Strontium Carb. if it becomes a chronic weak ankle.

❑ Fractures: first Arnica; afterwards when the bone is set, Symphytum.

Boxing:

❑ Shock: Arnica 10M.

❑ Anticipation anxiety before fight: Gelsemium 30C.
❑ Black eye: symphytum (#1), Ledum, Arnica.
❑ Contusions: Arnica, Ruta if periosteum is involved.
❑ Finger-hand injuries: Hypericum for nerve ending involvement with tingling and sharp pains; Hypericum for fractures.
❑ Contusions of head: Arnica 10M; Nat. Sulph. is a back-up; if there are convulsions after the trauma: Cicuta.
❑ Nasal bleeding: Arnica, Ferrum Phos., Vipera; put some Ferrum Phos on a tampon with gauze soaked in the solution.
❑ Cramps in calves: take Cuprum 200C before the fight.
❑ Blow over the heart: Arnica for the shock, Cactus 200C if there is a feeling of constriction.

Football:

❑ Sprains and strains: Rhus Tox., Ruta for acute; Strontium Carb. for chronic sequelae.
❑ Kicks and bruises on soft parts: Arnica before the game; Rhus Tox., Conium, Ruta.
❑ Synovitis: Ruta.
❑ Dislocation, subluxation: Rhus Tox. and Arnica.
❑ Contusions: from shock by colliding against another helmet, Arnica.
❑ Tendinitis: Ruta, Anacardium, Rhus Tox.

Tennis, ice skating, volley ball, soccer:

❑ Muscular exertion, sprains and strains: Arnica, Rhus Tox.
❑ Direct blow on the head: Arnica, Nat. Sulph.
❑ Blow on the leg, from raquet or kick: Ruta.
❑ Sunstroke: Glonoin.
❑ Tennis ball in eye: Symphytum, Hypericum.
❑ Tennis elbow: Ruta, Rhus Tox., Bellis Perennis.
❑ Injury in genital area: Arnica, Hypericum.
❑ Knee injury: Ruta.

Rock and mountain climbing:

❑ Frost bite and cold exposure: Agaricus #1.

❑ Altitude sickness: Coca and Carbo Vegetalis. These remedies are excellent for tourists visiting States like New Mexico and Colorado, while experiencing difficulties adjusting to the altitude, causing headaches, shortness of breath and extreme fatigue. They should start taking Carbo Veg. or Coca a couple of days before departure.

❑ Sunburn and sunstroke: Cantharis for sunburn, Glonoin for the consequences of sunstroke (dehydration, headaches).

SECTION THREE

MATERIA MEDICA OF MUSCULO-SKELETAL DISEASES

☛ **NOTE:** This Materia Medica is intended to help with "Musculoskeletal Diseases and Homeopathy." Therefore, characteristics and main indications refer mainly to the above class of illnesses. One exception has been made. Because of the importance of mental symptoms, whenever possible, the psychological characteristics of the remedy are noted. Text printed in **fat caps** means that the characteristic is outspoken and needs to be given more value than others in selecting the remedy. It is my hope that this "abbreviated Materia Medica" will lead to serious study for further exploration.

ACTAEA RACEMOSA (CIMICIFUGA)

KEYWORD: Arthritis of the **big** joints (Caulophyllum of the small joints).

PSYCHIC CHARACTERISTICS:
This is a patient (mainly female) with a **hysteric-rheumatic** constitution: often both entities alternate. **Loquacious** and incoherent, jumping from one subject to another. Deep sadness and gloom with **marked hypochondria**. Fear of becoming crazy and of death.

MUSCULOSKELETAL SYMPTOMS:
Sharp shooting neuralgic pains; strong muscle pains, aggravated by physical exercise; tenderness in the **first three lumbar** vertebrae; cramp-like **spasmodic** pains with stiffness.

AGGRAVATED:
- **during menses**
- by emotions
- by cold-humid weather

IMPROVED:
- by eating
- hot applications

MAIN CLINICAL INDICATIONS:
Osteo arthritis of the big joints (Hip).
Labor pains with severe "back breaking pains".
Intercostal rheumatism.

ACTEA SPICATA

KEYWORD: affinity for the **small** joints, especially in **men.**

MUSCULOSKELETAL SYMPTOMS: stiffness, paralytic pain and weakness in hands, tender to touch.

AGGRAVATED:
- at night

IMPROVED:
- in mornings

CLINICAL INDICATIONS:
Inflammatory arthritis of small joints (hand-feet).

AESCULUS HIPPOCASTANUM

KEYNOTE: Major hip remedy (#1).

PSYCHIC CHARACTERISTICS:
Tendency to **hypochondria** and sadness; often very bad disposition with **irritability**.

MUSCULOSKELETAL SYMPTOMS:
Sensation of **fullness** and heaviness, pulsating pains, formications. Sacrum feels as if dislocated, pain goes from sacrum to the hip; **weakness** in SI joints. Feeling that the lower back will break.

AGGRAVATED:
- **by rising from a seat**

- standing position
- waking up in the morning

IMPROVED:
- by prolonged movement
- by fresh air
- by cold baths

MAIN CLINICAL INDICATIONS:
Great affinity for the hips and the sacro-ilical joints.
Sciatica.
Gouty rheumatism of fore arm.

AGARICUS

KEYNOTE: twitches of the muscles (fibrillations, fasciculations).

PSYCHIC SYMPTOMS: **difficulties in comprehension**, irritable and depressed with **trembling;** fears of ghosts and dreaming of dead people; children alternate between silly, foolish behavior and depression; uncoordinated, backwards children.

MUSCULOSKELETAL SYMPTOMS: burning itching, alternating hot and cold pain sensations along the spine, "as if being pricked by thousand needles;" creeping, crawling sensations; electrical like pains through any part of the body; extreme sensitivity and tingling of the spine; back and neck feel dislocated.

AGGRAVATED:
- **intellectual activity**
- after sex
- after cold air and drinking cold water
- before storms (Rhododendron, Phos.)

IMPROVED:
- **by slow physical exercise** (yoga, Tai Chi)
- at sundown

MAIN CLINICAL INDICATIONS:
#1 for **frostbite**
#1 for Raynaud's Disease
#1 for twitching muscles (Tic Douloureux)
#1 for DT 's in alcoholic

AMMONIUM MURIATICUM

KEYNOTE: major sciatica remedy.

PSYCHIC CHARACTERISTICS:
Irritable in the morning; wants to cry but can't; fear of darkness; worse consolation.

MUSCULOSKELETAL SYMPTOMS:
Sensation of contracted muscles and tendons, too short (Caust., Nat.-m).

AGGRAVATED:
- by cold
- between 2-4 a.m.
- **sitting position**

IMPROVED:
- by fast walking
- by heat

MAIN CLINICAL INDICATIONS:
Sciatica.

Sacro-lumbar pain, especially at night.

ANTHRACINUM

KEYNOTE: hypersensitivity to the least touch.

MUSCULOSKELETAL SYMPTOMS:
Induration of inflammation, **intense burning feeling.**

MAIN CLINICAL INDICATIONS:
Boils, subungual abscesses, panaritium.

ANTIMONIUM CRUDUM

KEYNOTE: tongue looks **pasty** (thick, white coat).

PSYCHIC SYMPTOMS:
Children are like Chamomile children--hot-tempered, crying all the time except they **don't want to be carried or touched**! They do not bear being questioned or looked at. Adults are very **sentimental**, easily moved; they sulk, **love sickness**; pathological love lives (they follow stars around); end stage is often a loathing of life with suicidal depression.

MUSCULOSKELETAL SYMPTOMS:
Thickened skin due to overuse and pressure.

AGGRAVATED:
- by cold water
- by overeating of vinegar, pickles and acid foods
- by wine (Zinc, China)

- by touch and **consolation**

IMPROVED:
- by warm applications

MAIN CLINICAL INDICATIONS:
Corny and hard warts.
Calluses and corns and bonions.

APIS MELLIFICA

KEYNOTE: #1 for **hives**.

PSYCHIC SYMPTOMS:
Very **jealous** (Queen bee!); apathy or very attentive, irritable and suspicious.

MUSCULOSKELETAL SYMPTOMS:
Burning, **stinging**, wandering pains.

> ☛ **Note:** ❑ **burning and stinging : Apis**
> ❑ **burning and itching: Sulphur**
> ❑ **burning and sore: Causticum**

AGGRAVATED:
- **by heat**
- 4-6 p.m.
- by touch, even slight

IMPROVED:
- by cold, fresh air
- by abundant urination

MAIN INDICATIONS:
Acute inflammations (Bell.) Note: Chronic inflammations: Bryonia

ARNICA MONTANA

KEYNOTE: sportsman remedy #1.

PSYCHIC CHARACTERISTICS:
Stubborn, irritable persons, want to be alone. **Fear of being approached or touched when in pain.**

MUSCULOSKELETAL SYMPTOMS:
Sensation that the **bed is too hard**; sensation of a beat-up feeling, "as if a truck drove over them;" they can be in shock and say: "there is nothing wrong with me, I have no pain." Sore, **bruised** feeling.

AGGRAVATED:
- **by touch** (fear of being touched!)
- by the least exertion
- by cold-dampness
- by jolts and jars

IMPROVED:
- by hot applications
- by laying on back, head lower

MAIN INDICATIONS:
Trauma, contusion and shock.
Nws trauma.
Physical overexertion; muscular strain when overlifting.
Major gout remedy.
Complicated fractures. First remedy when **fracture**.

ARSENICUM ALBUM

KEYNOTE: **mental restlessness** with extreme **prostration;** body pains better with heat, head pains better with cold.

PSYCHIC SYMPTOMS:
Averse to amusement, brooding, disconted, gloom, grief, dwells on past disagreeable events, indifference to business and pleasure; biggest **"pest"**: "nothing is going to help him;" **very tidy**; very anxious about their health and fear of contamination; vain, capricious and true **hypochondriacs**.

MUSCULOSKELETAL SYMPTOMS:
Sensation of **intense burning** like hot coles, but relieved by heat!

AGGRAVATED:
- **between 1-3 a.m.**
- by thought of food
- **by cold (except headaches!)**

IMPROVED:
- by **heat**
- by warm drinks
- by changing position

MAIN CLINICAL INDICATIONS:
Shingles.
Panaritium.
Dry gangrene.
D.T.
Ascending paralysis (Conium)-Muscular atrophy.
Sciatica.

AURUM METALLICUM

KEYNOTE: constantly **dwelling on suicide**.

PSYCHIC SYMPTOMS:
Restless, always in a hurry and pacing the floor and say nothing; **severe depression with suicidal thoughts** combined with **anger**; despair about financial loss (Ars.); deep guilt and loneliness, especially after the loss of a "loved one;" they lost the "sunshine in their life:" desires death, **loathing of life**, they lost all value in life.

MUSCULOSKELETAL SYMPTOMS:
Boring, sharp pains in bones; great sensitivity to pain (Cham., Kali Carb.).

AGGRAVATED:
- by full moon, in evening
- by **financial loss or loss of a loved one**
- in winter

IMPROVED:
- by **sun-light**, in summer
- by walking in fresh air
- from music

MAIN CLINICAL INDICATIONS:
Tennis elbow.
Periostitis and osteitis.
Chronic gout.

BELLADONNA

KEYNOTE: "a pool of blood" (intense vascular congestion, hot-red, swollen).

PSYCHIC SYMPTOMS:
"Are angels when well, devils when sick"; very forgetful what they are doing.

MUSCULOSKELETAL SYMPTOMS:
Pains start and disappear quickly; **pulsing, throbbing** and **burning pains;** sharp, violent character of pathology; sensation that back is going to break.

AGGRAVATED:
- by **jolts**, jarring
- by cold
- around 9 p.m. and 3 p.m.

IMPROVEMENT:
- by bending backwards
- rest

MAIN INDICATIONS:
Articular inflammations.
Spasmodic phenomenons.
Lumbago.
Right laterality.

BELLIS PERENNIS

KEYNOTE: **deeper acting** Arnica, "gardener's remedy", dissolves ecchymoses.

MUSCULOSKELETAL SYMPTOMS:
Bruised feeling from over exertion.

AGGRAVATED:
- by touch
- by sudden cooling

IMPROVED:
- by cold (<> of Rhus tox!)
- by continued movement

MAIN INDICATIONS:
Tennis elbow.
Ecchymoses.
Muscular fatigue.
Cystic tumors after trauma (Conium).
Note: take Bellis in morning as it would give insomnia.

BENZOICUM ACIDUM

KEYNOTE: **urine smells like horse's urine**.

PSYCHIC SYMPTOMS:
Forget words while writing; sadness.

MUSCULOSKELETAL SYMPTOMS:
Pains change quickly from place to place (**fleeting);** feeling of cold sacrum.

AGGRAVATED:
- by weather changes
- **by cold air**
- by movement

IMPROVED:
- by heat
- **by abundant urine loss**

CLINICAL INDICATIONS:
Gout.
Arthritis of knee.

BRYONIA ALBA

KEYNOTE: pain experienced with the **slightest** movement; everything about Bry. is **dry**.

PSYCHIC SYMPTOMS:
Angry person, wants to be left alone (due to pain, aggravated by slightest movement); intolerance to contradiction.

MUSCULOSKELETAL SYMPTOMS:
Fierce, **immobilizing pains**; persistent pain under the left shoulder blade.

AGGRAVATED:
- by **slightest movement** (as much as moving of eyebrows!)
- around 9 p.m.

- by deep inspiration
- by light pressure

IMPROVED:
- by rest
- by **strong** pressure
- by lying on the painful side (it prevents the motion of the affected part)

CLINICAL INDICATIONS:
Predominantly **right-sided**.
Acute rheumatic arthritis.
Strong anti-inflammatory action in muscular rheumatism.
Whiplash (neck is frozen, does not want to be touched!).
Broken bones (Arn., Symph.).

CALCAREA CARBONICUM

KEYNOTE: **5 F's**: flabby, fat, fair, fears, faint.

PSYCHIC SYMPTOMS:
Very sensitive to **sad news** and music; very sympathetic and feeling **responsible for everything** and everybody; down to earth and practical; they feel overwhelmed by their worry and work. But there can be vehemence in their character, not only dullness. **Cerebral slowness**. Inaptitude for mathematics. Terrified of going insane.

MUSCULOSKELETAL SYMPTOMS:
Sacro-lumbar pains which hinder in getting up from sitting position. Stiffness of limbs when starting to move.

AGGRAVATED:
- by **cold (water, climate, etc.)**
- by exertion

IMPROVED:
- by dry weather

CLINICAL INDICATIONS:
Osteomalacie.
Osteoporosis (Calc. p).
Rickets.
Gout.

CALCAREA FLUORICA

KEYNOTE: acts on **bones** and **ligaments** (indicated in ptosis of the organs and laxness of ligaments); chronic of Ruta and Rhus Tox. (when the latter palliates).

PSYCHIC SYMPTOMS:
Methodical people, well organized but preoccupied with money.

MUSCULOSKELETAL SYMPTOMS:
Deformed bones, poor enamel in teeth. Often skoliosis present.

AGGRAVATED:
- by rest
- in beginning of movement

IMPROVED:
- by heat
- by frictions

CLINICAL INDICATIONS:
#1 for bone spurs or **exostoses**.
Bone tumors.
Tooth caries.
Repeated sprains.

CALCAREA PHOSPHORICA

KEYNOTE: causality is a combination of grief-overwork-excitement or many triggering factors at the same time.

PSYCHIC SYMPTOMS:
Fatigued by mental work, easily overwhelmed by stress.
Poor memory, rely on their intuition and enthusiasm.
Sentimental and easily moved.

MUSCULOSKELETAL SYMPTOMS:
Formication, very localized pains and locus dolendi on the long bones.

AGGRAVATED:
- by **change of weather**
- by thinking of his pains

IMPROVED:
- by heat

CLINICAL INDICATIONS:
#1 for **osteoporosis**.
Growing problems.
Caries.
#1 for growing pains in children.
Slow healing fractures (Symph.).

#1 for osteomyelitis.
#1 for osteogenesis imperfecta.
People with weak backs who are used to lift weights.

CAULOPHYLLUM

KEYNOTE: **small joints** are affected with at the same time complaints of female sexual system.

PSYCHIC SYMPTOMS:
Nervous personality, hysterical, and fearful.

MUSCULOSKELETAL SYMPTOMS:
Inflammation of the small articulations of hand and feet, **constantly changing** from place to place.

AGGRAVATED:
- by cold and draft

IMPROVED:
- by heat

CLINICAL INDICATIONS:
Rheumatism of small joints.

CAUSTICUM

KEYNOTE: predominantly **right**-sided; arthritis symptoms **better on whet days!**

PSYCHIC SYMPTOMS:
Very sensitive to the "wrongs" in the world; they can be sarcastic and revolting; they are sensitive and **idealistic**; easily disappointed; go through messy relationships with a lot of fighting. **Contradictory** personality.

MUSCULOSKELETAL SYMPTOMS:
Burning and soreness; burning, drawing pains, "as if the parts are too tight."; feeling of constriction.

AGGRAVATIONS:
- **by cold dry winds** (Patient needs a hat)
- around 3-4 a.m.
- by thinking of his complaints

IMPROVED:
- by **humidity** (Caust. is a dry remedy)
- by strong pressure

CLINICAL INDICATIONS:
#2 for torti collis (#1 is Lachnanthes).
#1 for **Bell's palsy**.
#1 for **Carpal tunnel syndrome**.
#1 for Dupuytren.
Chorea.
Writer's cramp.
Local paralysis (vocal chords, tongue, eyelids, etc.).
Bechterew.
Chronic rheumatism.
Coccydynia.
Maxillary arthritis.

☛NOTE: 3 top rheumatic remedies are: Sulphur, Rhus Tox and Caust.

CICUTA

KEYNOTE: **anti-convulsive** of the nervous system.

PSYCHIC SYMPTOMS:
Suspicious, melancholic, tearful, very forgetful, even for his own name; anxious for future.

MUSCULOSKELETAL SYMPTOMS:
Intense convulsions throughout the entire body **beginning in head** with rigidity in neck

AGGRAVATED:
- by touch and noise
- from frights

IMPROVED:
- by heat and rest

MAIN CLINICAL INDICATIONS:
Epilepsy.
Tetanus.
Chorea.

COLCHICUM

KEYNOTE: hypersensitive to odors, especially the smell of eggs causing nausea and general aggravation of symptoms.

PSYCHIC SYMPTOMS:
Irritable during pains, weak memory.

NEUROMUSCULAR SYMPTOMS: sensation of painful electrical vibrations, erratic, violent pains. The patient dreads the presence of anyone near him for fear of touching him.

AGGRAVATED:
- by **slightest movement** (Bry.) [opposite of Rhus Tox.]
- by change of weather, in **autumn**
- by cold-dampness (Rhus Tox.)

IMPROVED:
- by rest and heat

CLINICAL INDICATIONS:
Acute gout (Urt. Ur., Ledum).
Gouty rheumatism with arthritic nodosity.

COLOCYNTHIS

KEYNOTE: pain improves by **bending forward and doubling over;** predominantly **left-sided**.

PSYCHIC SYMPTOMS:
Restless and **easily offended**; they don't want to hear questions; irritable and agitated.

NEUROMUSCULAR SYMPTOMS:
Cutting, stabbing and pinching pain, comes and goes quickly, leg feels lame and weak.

AGGRAVATED:
- by being yelled at (**indignation**)
- in morning
- 4 p.m.
- by rest

IMPROVED:
- **bending forward and doubling over**
- **by strong pressure**
- by being alone

CLINICAL INDICATIONS:
Sciatica: pain with numbness.
Cramping pains with lumbago and torticollis.

CUPRUM METALLICUM

KEYNOTE: massive spasms, > **with drinking a sip of cold water**.

PSYCHIC SYMPTOMS:
Hypersensitive people, very anxious and fearful; incoherent loquacity in delirium; **bored stiff if idle**; they are never content to do nothing.

MUSCULOSKELETAL SYMPTOMS:
Violent cramps **starting in extremities**; fingers and toes cramp up, **thumb is flexed** inside the clenched fist; begins and ends suddenly; **blue fingers**.

AGGRAVATED:
- by touch
- inhaling cold air
- at night and new moon

IMPROVED:
- **by drinking sips of cold water**

MAIN CLINICAL INDICATIONS:
Epileptic disorders.
Foot and leg cramps in elderly (Mag.-p, Calc. carb.).
Contracture of muscles and localized muscular paralysis.

DIOSCOREA

Keynote: pains improve by **bending backwards**.

NEUROMUSCULAR SYMPTOMS:
Violent, cramping, cutting pain, radiating; colicky pain; shifts suddenly to different parts.

AGGRAVATED:
- by **bending forward**
- in evening and night
- when lying down

IMPROVED:
- by **bending backwards** or standing straight

CLINICAL INDICATIONS:
Sciatica.
Knee pains.

FERRUM METALLICUM

KEYNOTE: **3 F's**: Flushed, Feeble, Faint.

PSYCHIC SYMPTOMS:
Feeble, incapable of prolonged efforts; cold sensitive; blushes easily but at rest is always pale.

MUSCULOSKELETAL SYMPTOMS:
Pulsating and hammering pains; easy bruising.

AGGRAVATED:
- by **cold**
- by immobility or moving quickly
- by excitement

IMPROVED:
- by moving or walking **slowly** (Puls.)
- by fresh air

MAIN CLINICAL INDICATIONS:
Frozen shoulder and hip rheumatism.
Lumbago.

GNAPHALIUM

KEYNOTE: elective action on trigeminus nerve and sciatic nerve (**Right-sided**).

MUSCULOSKELETAL SYMPTOMS:
Pain alternating with numbness, articular stiffness; intense neuralgic pains along the nerve like Colocynth.

AGGRAVATED:
- by walking

IMPROVED:
- by sitting with legs folded

CLINICAL INDICATIONS:
Right-sided sciatica.
Acute gout.
Lumbago.

GRAPHITES

KEYNOTE: is the Sulphur of women, **cracked skin**.

PSYCHIC SYMPTOMS:
Very **indecisive**, moody and obstinent, low sex drive (Sep.), sensitive to music, sensitive to wrongs in this world, wants justice (Caust.).

MUSCULOSKELETAL SYMPTOMS:
Thick, brittle deformed nails; itching and burning.

AGGRAVATED:
- by cold-dampness
- by heat of bed
- around **menopause**
- by music which makes her cry

IMPROVED:
- in evening
- after eating
- in fresh air, wrapped up warmly

MAIN CLINICAL INDICATIONS:
Periungual warts.
Nail disorders.
Chronic gout.

GUAIACUM

KEYNOTE: craves apples; predominantly **left-sided**.

PSYCHIC SYMPTOMS:
Depressed and sad people with a loss of memory for names.

MUSCULOSKELETAL SYMPTOMS:
Burning pain with a feeling of **contraction**: muscles and tendons feel too short; mainly in wrist and ankles..

AGGRAVATED:
- by touch and **heat**
- by the least movement

IMPROVED:
- by cold applications (Ledum, Puls., Lac.can.)

CLINICAL INDICATIONS:
Carpal tunnel syndrome (Caust.).
Dupuytren's contracture (Caust.).
P.C.E.
Torticollis and lumbago.

HEKLA LAVA

KEYNOTE: exostose remedy.
MAIN CLINICAL INDICATIONS:
Bone spurs (Calc-f).
Exostose of the jaw bone. Use 6C if not painful, 30C if painful.

HYPERICUM PERFORATUM

KEYNOTE: is a remedy for **nerve endings**.

PSYCHIC SYMPTOMS:
Depressed after a trauma; tea stimulates the brain.

NEUROMUSCULAR SYMPTOMS:
Sharp, shooting radiating pain along the nerve, burning and tingling.

AGGRAVATED:
- by being **jolted** and by touch
- by fog, cold, dampness

IMPROVED:
- by bending the head backwards

CLINICAL INDICATIONS:
#1 for dog bites and animal bites and insect sting.
#1 for puncture wounds (spinal taps, biopsies, allergy shots).
Laceration of a nail.
Amputation or phantom pains.
Fall on tail bone.
Injuries to the spine and #1 for brachial neuralgia.

KALI BICHROMICUM

KEYNOTE: pain in **small spots** (Ign., Onosm.); alternation between rheumatism and intestinal disorders.

PSYCHIC SYMPTOMS:
Indifferent with an aversion for intellectual work.

NEURO MUSCULAR SYMPTOMS:
Pains **come and go quickly**, very localized, relieved by the pressure of a finger; wandering stitchy pains.

AGGRAVATED:
- by **cold**
- by undressing
- between 2-3 a.m.

IMPROVED:
- by heat

CLINICAL INDICATIONS:
Left-sided sciatica.
Pains in heels (talalgia).
Coccyodynia.
Lumbago.

KALI CARBONICUM

KEYNOTE: **backaches preceding the menstrual cycle; < 2-5 a.m.;** edema of upper eyelid.

PSYCHIC SYMPTOMS:
Strong sense of duty, very **dogmatic** and "by the book;" likes routine; many issues around **control** with narrow, rigid thinking; tendency to minimize his symptoms, he denies his feelings; maintains a tight control over expressing his emotions; he is **hypersensitive** to noise, touch and draft; easily absent-minded.

NEUROMUSCULAR SYMPTOMS:
Sharp, stabbing and stitching pains, **relieved by movement** (Rhus Tox); feeling of **weakness**, "as if the legs are going to give away;" extending to tigh.

AGGRAVATED:
- by **cold**
- by sleeping on affected side (<> of Bry.)
- sitting

IMPROVED:
- by heat
- by **movement**

CLINICAL INDICATIONS:
Sacro-ilical syndrome, esp. on the right (Aesc.).
Lumbago, especially premenstrual; also after injury.
Wandering arthritis.

KALI IODATUM

KEYNOTE: "rocking the head from side to side".

PSYCHIC SYMPTOMS:
Irritable, easily offended, ill-humored.

MUSCULOSKELETAL SYMPTOMS:
Sharp, deep pains.

AGGRAVATED:
- by heat (<> of Rhus Tox.!)
- **at night, after patient has gone to bed**
- from sunset to sunrise
- lying on affected side

IMPROVED:
- by movement
- by exposure to **cool air**

MAIN CLINICAL INDICATIONS:
Sciatica with all the symptoms of Rhus Tox. except improvement with heat.
Gout.
Acute and chronic rheumatism.

KALMIA LATIFOLIA

KEYNOTE: after the pain leaves, **numbness follows.**

MUSCULOSKELETAL SYMPTOMS:
Rheumatic pains move quickly from place to place (Bry., Kali Bich., Puls.); pains **move downwards**, especially from shoulder to elbow and wrist, with a feeling of great weakness; electrical neuralgic pains, following nerve paths from the center outwards.

AGGRAVATED:
- **by moving**
- in first half of the night and 2 p.m.

IMPROVED:
- while **eating**
- in overcast weather

CLINICAL INDICATIONS:
Tic douloureux...
#1 for **trigeminus neuralgia** (Right side; left: Spigelia).
Sciatica and lumbago.
#1 for **rheumatic fever**.
Bechterew.
Herpes Zoster.

LACHNANTHES

KEYNOTE: **right-sided** laterality.

PSYCHIC SYMPTOMS:
Very loquacious with red face and fiery eyes.

MUSCULOSKELETAL SYMPTOMS:
Sensation of pinched nerve in neck; **painful stiffness** of the neck with head curbed to the side.

AGGRAVATED:
- from 1-2 a.m.

CLINICAL INDICATIONS:
#1 for **Torti collis**
Rheumatism of neck

LEDUM PALUSTRE

KEYNOTE: is a combination of Arnica and Hypericum.

PSYCHIC SYMPTOMS:
Angry people preferring to live by themselves.

MUSCULOSKELETAL SYMPTOMS:
Sharp pains which begin in feet and **move upwards** (<> of Kalmia).

AGGRAVATED:
- by local heat
- by movement
- by pressure

IMPROVED:
- by **cold** applications (the patient puts his feet in ice water)
- by emission of red sand-like urine (Lyc.)

CLINICAL INDICATIONS:
#1 for wounds caused by a sharp object (wounds are apt to become cold; puffiness, little bleeding).
#1 for "black" eye.
Insect bites, mosquito bites, flea bites.
Gout of big toe.
Traumatic arthritis.
Remedy for old sinners, especially alcoholics (Nux-Vom., Sulph. Acid, Agnus Castus).

MAGNESIA PHOSPHORICA

KEYNOTE: Right-sided; main idea: against cramps.

PSYCHIC SYMPTOMS:
Nervous type talking incessantly about their crampy pains.

MUSCULOSKELETAL SYMPTOMS:
Crampy pains, suddenly coming up, changing quickly from place to place.

AGGRAVATED:
- by cold
- at night
- by overuse

IMPROVED:
- by **hot** water
- by leaning forward and **doubling up**; by pressure

CLINICAL INDICATIONS:
Sciatica.
Writer's cramp.
Player's cramp

MEDORRHINUM

KEYNOTE: improves at the seaside; craves oranges; sleeps in genu-pectoral position.

PSYCHIC SYMPTOMS:
Passionate, impulsive people, especially when it comes to sex. They **live in the fast lane:** sex, drugs and rock and roll. They have a fear of losing control (Kali Carb, Calc. carb.), fear of going crazy. People with **unstable vitality** (cyclothymic).

MUSCULOSKELETAL SYMPTOMS:
Trembling feeling throughout the body; burning pain along the spine; heels and soles are very ticklish; burning heat in hands and feet; alternating pains from left to right to left (Lac.can.).

AGGRAVATED:
- by alcohol
- during the daytime
- by thinking of his pains
- at stagnant waters (swamps)

IMPROVED:
- **from sundown to sunset**
- in dampness
- **at the seaside**
- lying on stomach
- by continuous movement

CLINICAL INDICATIONS:
Chronic rheumatism.
Talalgia.

NATRUM CARBONICUM

KEYNOTE: weak ankle remedy; aggravated symptoms by the least change of weather.

PSYCHIC SYMPTOMS:
Very **depressed** and hypochondriac. Headaches from intellectual work. They do not like physical or mental work. Very **melancholic** and sensitive to music. They withdraw when grieving.

MUSCULOSKELETAL SYMPTOMS:
Trembling and sweating with their pains.

AGGRAVATED:
- **by least change of weather (Merc.Sol.)**
- by playing the piano
- by sex and exhaustion
- by storms

IMPROVED:
- by motion

CLINICAL INDICATIONS:
Recurrent sprained ankles.
Fragility of joints (Calc.-f).

NATRUM SULFURICUM

KEYNOTE: right-sided remedy.

PSYCHIC SYMPTOMS:
Depressed and slow intellectually, especially concentration.

MUSCULOSKELETAL SYMPTOMS:
General feeling of **stiffness** and sharp pains.

AGGRAVATED:
- **cold-dampness**
- in spring
- at seaside
- by sun (headaches especially)

IMPROVED:
- by **dry weather**
- by changing position and slow progressive motion (Rhus Tox)

CLINICAL INDICATIONS:
#1 for **nws head trauma** (#2 Arnica).
Trauma to cervical and thoracic spine.
Acute coxarthritis.

PHYTOLACCA

KEYNOTE: Phytolacca is between Rhus Tox and Bryonia.

PSYCHIC SYMPTOMS:
Easily depressed, convinced they are going to die.

MUSCULOSKELETAL SYMPTOMS:
The pain **forces the patient to move but movement does not relieve**; has **stiffness** like Rhus Tox; sharp electrical nerve pains, abruptly changing places.

AGGRAVATED:
- at night and in **damp** weather
- with movement (with desire to move)
- by lying on the right side

IMPROVED:
- by dry weather

CLINICAL INDICATIONS:
Sciatica (L4-L5).
Talalgia.
TMJ.
Frozen shoulder.

PLUMBUM METALLICUM

KEYNOTE: **immense thirst**; feeling of a tight band tied around the leg (in claudicatio).

PSYCHIC SYMPTOMS:
Slow intelligence, can't find the right word; taciturn and indifferent; **melancholic** and religious mania; inclination to cheat and deceive; restless sleepers.

MUSCULOSKELETAL SYMPTOMS:
Constrictive, violent pains; shooting neuralgic pains; paralysis of the extensor muscles with atrophy.

AGGRAVATED:
- by movement
- by superficial touch

IMPROVED:
- **by strong pressure**
- **by doubling up** (Mag. Phos.)

MAIN CLINICAL INDICATIONS:
Wrist drop and foot drop.

Polio.
Chronic sciatica.
Muscular atrophy.

PULSATILLA

KEYNOTE: one-sided remedy, **changeable** symptoms.

PSYCHIC SYMPTOMS:
Very **moody** with ups and downs, easily impressed, crying with laughing in the next minute, brooding, **shy**, extreme mother instincts; they love and **look for consolation**; down to earth; dread for men; capricious, docile, **easily offended**.

MUSCULOSKELETAL SYMPTOMS:
Pain is **erratic**, electrical discharges, symptoms mainly located on one side.

AGGRAVATED:
- at twilight **(5 p.m.)**
- by heat and in a hot room

IMPROVED:
- by slowly walking
- by being **outside**
- by cold compresses

CLINICAL INDICATIONS:
Wandering pain in Rheumatoid Arthritis.
Gonarthritis.

RADIUM BROMATUM

KEYNOTE: resembles Puls. and Rhus Tox; Radium has the greatest affinity for the **cartilaginous and bony part** of the articulation; Rhus Tox. more for the sheath of the muscles.

PSYCHIC SYMPTOMS:
Depressed individuals, fearful of loneliness and that something bad is going to happen to them.

MUSCULOSKELETAL SYMPTOMS:
Sensation of **general burning** with desire of fresh air; electrical sudden pains with sensation of stiffness and lame feeling.

AGGRAVATED:
- when **movement starts** (Rhus Tox)
- at night

IMPROVED:
- by **continued movement**
- in open air
- by heat

CLINICAL INDICATIONS:
Lumbo-sacral rheumatism.
Gout.

RANUNCULUS BULBOSUS

KEYNOTE: vesicular eruptions with a **characteristic bluish color**.

PSYCHIC: irritable and fearful of being alone

MUSCULOSKELETAL SYMPTOMS:
Shooting piercing pains in the **intercostal spaces**

AGGRAVATED:
- in evening
- by pressure
- by change in weather
- by movement

CLINICAL INDICATIONS:
Intercostal neuralgia (Herpes Zoster).
Herpes Zoster of the Vth nerve.
Post-zonal neuralgias.
Rib pains.

RHODODENDRON

KEYNOTE: aggravated when a **storm is approaching.**

PSYCHIC SYMPTOMS:
Nervous individual who is very fearful of storms (because patient aggravates before the storm and is relieved after the storm breaks).

MUSCULOSKELETAL SYMPTOMS:
Searing zigzag pains, deep pains with feeling of paralysis.

AGGRAVATED:
- by **stormy weather** (Dulc.)
- by rest

IMPROVED:
- after the storm
- by motion

CLINICAL INDICATIONS:
Rheumatism set off by storms.
Trigeminus neuralgia.
Lumbago.
Torticollis.

RHUS TOXICODENDRON

KEYNOTE: called the **"rusty hinge"** and the **"human barometer"**.

PSYCHIC SYMPTOMS:
Great anxiety at night preventing them from sleep, with great physical restlessness.

MUSCULOSKELETAL SYMPTOMS:
Outspoken articular **stiffness** with bruised feeling and feeling of luxation, feeling of cold water thrown on the body; burning, drawing and shooting pains.

AGGRAVATED:
- by rest
- at **night**
- by beginning of the movement and when the patient is tired (aggravation after long continued movement)
- by **dampness**
- by change of weather and after the storm breaks

IMPROVED:
- **by continued movement, slow motion**
- by massage and manipulation
- by heat
- in dry hot weather
- **by changing position**

CLINICAL INDICATIONS:
Lumbago.
Sciatica.
Sprains and dislocations (Ruta).
Rheumatism resulting from or aggravated by dampness.
Muscular exertion.
#1 for Intercostal neuralgia.

RUTA GRAVEOLENS

KEYNOTE: is a combination of Rhus Tox and Arnica, active on **ligaments and periosteum**.

PSYCHIC SYMPTOMS:
Inclined to be ill-humored, melancholic and depressed.

MUSCULOSKELETAL SYMPTOMS:
A feeling of **contusion** and **stiffness**, especially of the limbs and articulations; heaviness of the limbs; digging pain of tendons

AGGRAVATED:
- by cold-dampness
- by lying down; there is a constant need for changing position

IMPROVED:
- by **motion**

- by changing position

CLINICAL INDICATIONS:
#1 for tennis elbow.
Carpal tunnel syndrome.
Frozen shoulder.
Dislocated joints or tendency to dislocate.
Chronic weak legs after back injury ("lame" feeling).
Achilles tendon lesion.
Sprains (#2 after Rhus Tox.).
Overuse of limbs.
NOTE: if Ruta palliates, go to Calc.-f!

SANGUINARIA CAN.

KEYNOTE: **right-sided** affinity.

PSYCHIC SYMPTOMS:
Debilitated and weak especially upon awakening; irritable and weak memory.

MUSCULOSKELETAL SYMPTOMS:
Burning pain with sensation of dry mucosae.

AGGRAVATED:
- at night
- on turning in bed and raising the arm
- periodically

IMPROVED:
- by sleep
- by lying on back

MAIN CLINICAL INDICATIONS:
Right frozen shoulder.
Lumbago.
Muscular rheumatism.

SECALE CORNUTUM

KEYNOTE: **skin feels cold to the touch, yet the patient cannot stand being covered.**

PSYCHIC SYMPTOMS:
Fear for dying, loss of memory after sex.

MUSCULOSKELETAL SYMPTOMS:
Intense burning, but entire surface of body is cold; formication.

AGGRAVATED:
- by **heat**
- by being covered

IMPROVED:
- by **cool places**
- after dinner

MAIN CLINICAL INDICATIONS:
Raynaud's Disease.
Dry gangrene (Ars.).

SEPIA

KEYNOTE: hormonal imbalance and prolaps remedy.

PSYCHIC SYMPTOMS:
Has the vehemence and irritability of Nux Vomica, despondency of Pulsatilla or the apathy of Phosporus **intensified**; could care less if she ever had sex; only **sex out of obligation**; total **indifference,** even to loved ones; dead emotionally, their motto is, “I don’t care;” poor memory and concentration, < premenstrual; they have a **sharp tongue** and are not sympathetic to others; an urge to clean premenstrual; taciturn and burnt out feeling; excited by thunderstorms; loss of motherly instincts, aloof and detached; hates to tell what ails her.

MUSCULOSKELETAL SYMPTOMS:
Sensation of heaviness and tugging pains in back and sacrum **(bearing down sensation)**; pains have a tendency to radiate to the lower back, cold feeling with chills.

AGGRAVATED:
- **by standing or rest**
- premenstrual

IMPROVED:
- **by strenuous exercise** (they are the ones who have to exercise to feel good, aerobics, jogging, dancing, etc.)

MAIN CLINICAL INDICATIONS:
Raynaud’s Disease #2 (Agaricus #1).
Chronic sciatica.
Articular laxity.

SILICEA

KEYNOTE: remedy for suppressed foot sweat.

PSYCHIC SYMPTOMS:
Lack of confidence but great courage; spineless, they believe everything what is said; lack of stamina; inability to stand up for themselves; children are **delicate,** picky in eating, clean and **orderly**; anticipation anxiety although when performing, they succeed.

MUSCULOSKELETAL SYMPTOMS:
Icy cold feeling, feeling of needles in tissues.

AGGRAVATED:
- by **mental and physical exertion**
- by exposure to cold and wind (they wear hats)

IMPROVED:
- by heat

MAIN CLINICAL INDICATIONS:
Boils, abscesses.
Panaritium.
Rachitis, osteomalacy.
Pott's disease and TB arthritis.

STAPHYSAGRIA

KEYNOTE: ailments from indignation (abuse, shame and suppressed anger).

PSYCHIC SYMPTOMS:
Easily offended, can't forget the past insults; preoccupied sexually but timid to the opposite sex, therefore tendency to **masturbation**; pathological desire to please; cannot tolerate injustice (Caust.); irrational resentment; the staph. woman does

not want to cry in front of others because they might suffer and she does not want to upset others; she will accept inconvenience and unjust acts; **resignation** becomes the most dominant feeling.

NEUROMUSCULAR SYMPTOMS:
Hypersensitivity physically and emotionally; nightly bone pains; sensation of itching stitches.

AGGRAVATED:
- by **anger**
- by touch
- at new moon

IMPROVED:
- by heat and rest

CLINICAL INDICATIONS:
Back pains since indignation
Pains after incised surgical wounds (**nws surgery #1**).

SULPHUR

KEYNOTE: "sticks his feet out of bed", he wants to uncover them; early morning diarrhea drives him out of bed; "all-gone" feeling in stomach around 11 a.m.

PSYCHIC SYMPTOMS:
Careless, emotional unstable and aversion to physical exercise; the ragged philosopher; **egotistic** and arrogant; leadership; sharp tongue; is feared and admired; **impulsive anger** with outbursts; **critical** of others but sensitive to criticism; loses interest quickly.

MUSCULOSKELETAL SYMPTOMS:
Burning and itching, throbbing pains (Bell.)

AGGRAVATED:
- by **heat and warmth of bed**
- by **water**
- around **11 a.m.** and 5 p.m.
- by wool and feathers (allergic)

IMPROVED:
- by **motion**
- by **dry weather**

MAIN CLINICAL INDICATIONS:
Lumbago.
Rheumatism (Rhus Tox. is complementary) anywhere in body.
TB arthritis.

SYMPHYTUM

KEYNOTE: **remarkable cure for fractures**.

MUSCULOSKELETAL SYMPTOMS:
Pains increase and decrease slowly; linear pains.

CLINICAL INDICATIONS:
Fractures: first give Arnica, once the bone is set, give Symphytum.
#1 for **black eye** (Ledum #2).
Osteoporosis.
Osteogenesis imperfecta.
Bone cancer (Hekla Lava).
Phantom pains.

TELLURIUM

KEYNOTE: affinity for **sacral plexus** and **sciatic nerve**.

MUSCULOSKELETAL SYMPTOMS:
Whole spine is **hypersensitive** to the least touch; pains appear and disappear suddenly; sharp, radiating pain; <C7-T5 and S1 zones).

AGGRAVATED:
- by touch and lying down on affected area

MAIN CLINICAL INDICATIONS:
Sciatica
Tailbone injury
Injuries to the spine (Nat. sulph., Agar., Hyper.)

URTICA URENS

KEYNOTE: **stinging**, **nettling** feeling.

MUSCULOSKELETAL DISEASES:
Prickly, stinging, burning itching.

AGGRAVATED:
- by cold applications of water
- by touch

CLINICAL INDICATIONS:
#1 for **gout,** removing the uric acid; in tincture, 10 drops BID

INDEX

A

B

C

D

E

F

G

H

I

P

Q

R

S

T

U

V

W

ORDERFORM

Pleasae send (   ) copy(ies) of the book

"Full OF LIFE"

How to Achieve and Maintain Peak Immunity

Unit price: $12.95
Postage: $3.00
New Mexico residents add 6.125% sales tax

Ship to:

Name: ______________________________

Street: ______________________________

City ______________ State ________ Zip: ________

Total purchase amount: $

Mastercard or VISA: Number: ______________________
Expiration date: ____________

Please send check or money order to:

FULL OF LIFE PUBL.
PO BOX 31025
SANTA FE, NM 87594

ORDERFORM

Pleasae send ( ) copy(ies) of the book

"HOW TO DINE LIKE THE DEVIL AND FEEL LIKE A SAINT"

Good-Bye To Guilty Eating

Unit price: $17.95
Postage: $3.00
New Mexico residents add 6.125% sales tax

Ship to:

Name: ____

Street: ____

City ________________________ State ____________ Zip: ____________

Total purchase amount: $

Mastercard or VISA: Number: ______________________
Expiration date: ____________

Please send check or money order to:

Full of Life Publishing
500 N. Guadalupe St. G441,
Santa Fe, NM 87501

ORDERFORM

Pleasae send ( ) copy(ies) of the book

"HUMAN CONDITION: CRITICAL"

Unit price: $12.95
Postage: $3.00
New Mexico residents add 6.125% sales tax

Ship to:

Name: ______________________________

Street: ______________________________

City ______________ State ______ Zip: ______

Total purchase amount: $

Mastercard or VISA: Number: ___________________________
Expiration date: _______________

Please send check or money order to:

Full of Life Publishing
500 N. Guadalupe St. G441,
Santa Fe, NM 87501